Metabolic Flexibility

How the Body Switches Between Fat and Glucose for Energy and Metabolic Health

Nathan Reed

PERENNIAL PUBLISHING

Published by Perennial Publishing

Paperback ISBN: 978-1-971996-42-4
Hardcover ISBN: 978-1-971996-43-1
E-book ISBN: 978-1-971996-44-8

Contents

Introduction

Metabolic signals are often the most visible elements of the system, and that visibility creates a sense of immediacy that is easily mistaken for understanding. Glucose values, fluctuations in energy, and patterns of hunger appear concrete and self-contained, presenting themselves as if they carry their own explanations. The act of observing these outputs can produce confidence that the system has been understood simply because it has been seen. This confidence emerges from the assumption that what is visible is also transparent, that the signal reveals not only that something has occurred but why it has occurred.

This assumption collapses a critical distinction between observation and explanation. A signal indicates that the system has produced an output, but it does not disclose the processes that generated that output. The underlying mechanisms remain distributed across multiple pathways, interacting across time and influenced by prior conditions that are not visible in the signal itself. Treating the signal as its own explanation removes these mechanisms from consideration, reducing a coordinated system to a single observable point.

Reestablishing this distinction is the first structural shift required for accurate interpretation. Observation identifies what has occurred, but explanation requires access to the processes that produced it. Signals are therefore positioned as outputs of the system rather than representations of its internal structure. They are endpoints of interaction, not descriptions of mechanism, and must be interpreted with reference to the system that produced them.

Metabolic outputs function as compressed representations of system behavior, integrating multiple upstream processes into a single observable form. A glucose value, for example, reflects the interaction of external input, absorption dynamics, distribution across tissues, cellular uptake, endogenous production, signaling coordination, and current demand. These processes are not visible independently within the signal; they are combined into a unified output that summarizes their collective effect. Compression allows the system to present complex behavior in a simplified form, but it obscures the structure that produced that behavior.

This compression introduces ambiguity into interpretation because the same output can arise from different underlying configurations. A single signal does not correspond to a single cause but to a range of possible interactions that converge at the point of observation. Without expanding the signal back into its contributing processes, interpretation remains incomplete. The signal provides evidence that something has occurred within the system, but it does not specify which processes were responsible or how they interacted.

Understanding signals as compressed outputs shifts interpretation away from direct reading and toward structural reconstruction. The task becomes identifying the processes that could have produced the observed output, recognizing that multiple pathways may contribute simultaneously. This reframing prevents signals from being treated as isolated explanations and instead positions them as summaries that require context and expansion to be understood.

Metabolic interpretation often isolates individual moments and treats them as complete units of meaning. A meal, a measurement, or a perceived shift in energy is framed as a discrete event with defined boundaries, suggesting that it can be understood independently of what precedes or follows it. This framing implies that the system begins and resolves within the moment of observation, allowing the event to be treated as both cause and outcome.

The system does not operate within these boundaries. Each observed moment is embedded within a continuous sequence of processes that extend beyond the event itself. Prior inputs influence current conditions, ongoing signaling shapes how the system responds, and substrate distribution reflects a history of previous interactions. The event is therefore a fragment of an ongoing process rather than a standalone occurrence. Its meaning cannot be determined without reference to the processes that surround it.

Interpreting events as fragments of continuous processes shifts the focus from isolated moments to sequences of interaction. The system is understood as operating across time, with each moment reflecting both past influences and current conditions. This perspective replaces event-based interpretation with process-based interpretation, where meaning is derived from continuity rather than from isolated observation.

The metabolic system operates as a continuous flow of energy redistribution, maintaining alignment between supply and demand without interruption. Energy demand persists across time, requiring supply to be adjusted continuously rather than activated intermittently. There are no points at which the system becomes inactive or transitions between discrete states of operation. Instead, it maintains a constant process of adjustment, modulating the contribution of different pathways to sustain continuity.

This continuous operation involves overlapping contributions from multiple substrates. Glucose and fat are both present and active to varying degrees, with their relative contributions shifting gradually in response to changes in availability, signaling, and demand. These shifts occur without abrupt transitions, forming gradients rather than discrete switches. The system remains in motion at all times, even when external conditions appear stable.

Within this framework, stability is not defined by the absence of change but by the coordination of ongoing adjustment. A stable system maintains alignment across its components as they continuously adapt to internal and external conditions. This redefines stability as a dynamic property, where continuity of function is preserved through coordinated movement rather than through static balance.

The meaning of any metabolic signal depends on the context in which it is produced. The same observable output can correspond to different underlying processes depending on the system's current state. This state is shaped by prior inputs, recent transitions, signaling conditions, substrate distribution, and the presence of constraints that influence how pathways interact. Context determines how inputs are processed and how outputs are generated, making it a central factor in interpretation.

Because the system carries forward the effects of prior activity, there is no reset between events. Each new condition emerges from the accumulation of previous conditions, creating a layered structure in which current behavior reflects both present and past influences. A signal observed in one context cannot be interpreted in the same way when that context differs, even if the observable output appears identical.

This dependency on context prevents signals from being interpreted in isolation. Meaning emerges from the interaction between the signal and the system state that produced it. Interpretation must therefore account for the configuration of the system at the time of observation, recognizing that outputs are conditional rather than absolute. Without this context, signals remain ambiguous and open to misinterpretation.

Metabolic behavior is governed by constraints rather than by preference or intention. The system does not select substrates based on goals or optimization but operates within the limits imposed by availability, access, signaling, and suppression. These constraints define which pathways are active, how strongly they contribute, and how they interact with one another. Outcomes emerge from these conditions rather than from deliberate selection.

Substrate dominance reflects the configuration of constraints at a given time. When glucose is readily available and supported by signaling conditions that promote its use, it becomes the dominant contributor. When access to stored energy increases and suppression is reduced, fat contribution expands. These shifts occur as a result of regulatory processes, not as expressions of choice. The system responds to conditions rather than directing them.

Understanding behavior as constraint-driven removes the need to assign intention to metabolic patterns. Outcomes are not chosen; they are enforced by the structure of the system and the conditions in which it operates. Interpretation must therefore focus on the constraints that shape behavior rather than on the appearance of the outcome itself.

Transitions within the metabolic system are continuous processes rather than discrete events. The redistribution of energy between substrates occurs through gradual changes in contribution, with glucose and fat remaining present at all times. There is no singular point at which one substrate replaces another. Instead, their relative contributions shift along a continuum, forming overlapping patterns of use.

This continuous redistribution reflects the system's constant adjustment to changing conditions. Small variations occur continuously, often below the threshold of visibility, while larger shifts become noticeable when the gradient of change increases. The system is therefore always in transition, even when it appears stable. What is observed as a transition is part of an ongoing process rather than a distinct event.

Recognizing transitions as continuous processes removes the concept of isolated switching moments. The system does not move between fixed states but maintains a constant flow of adjustment, where multiple processes overlap across time. Interpretation must therefore account for this continuity, understanding that all observed changes are part of an ongoing sequence rather than discrete shifts.

Metabolic signals are outputs of a coordinated system, not independent explanations of its behavior. These outputs compress multiple interacting processes into visible forms that require expansion to be understood. Events are fragments of continuous processes, and the system operates without discrete states or isolated transitions. Behavior is shaped by constraints, and signals acquire meaning only within the context of the system state in which they are produced.

This framework replaces event-based interpretation with system-based interpretation. The focus shifts from individual signals to the processes that generate them, from isolated moments to continuous sequences, and from assumed causes to interacting mechanisms. Interpretation becomes an examination of how the system functions across time rather than a reading of what it displays at a single point.

The metabolic system is therefore understood as a continuous, context-dependent structure in which all observable outputs reflect underlying coordination. Signals do not explain themselves, events do not stand alone, and outcomes do not arise from single inputs. Meaning emerges from the interaction of processes operating across time, and interpretation must follow that structure.

Dual-Fuel Mechanism

Energy use within the human metabolic system is often interpreted as if it were singular, as though the system operates on a single dominant substrate that defines its state at any given moment. This interpretation compresses a multi-pathway structure into a simplified model that cannot account for observed variability across time, condition, and demand. The system does not rely on a single fuel source. It is organized around the coexistence of multiple substrates, with glucose and fat representing the primary contributors to energy production under most conditions. These substrates are not sequential replacements for one another, nor are they arranged in a hierarchy of preference. They exist in parallel, embedded within a system that continuously evaluates availability, constraint, and demand.

Glucose and fat are present within the system at all times. Their presence is not conditional, even if their utilization is. Glucose circulates within the bloodstream, is stored in limited quantities as glycogen, and is continuously regulated through input, endogenous production, and cellular uptake. Fat exists primarily in stored form, distributed across adipose tissue, with a circulating component that becomes more prominent under certain conditions. Both substrates are accessible through established metabolic pathways, each with its own regulatory controls, enzymatic requirements, and rates of mobilization. The system maintains readiness for both pathways simultaneously, regardless of which substrate is currently dominant in energy production.

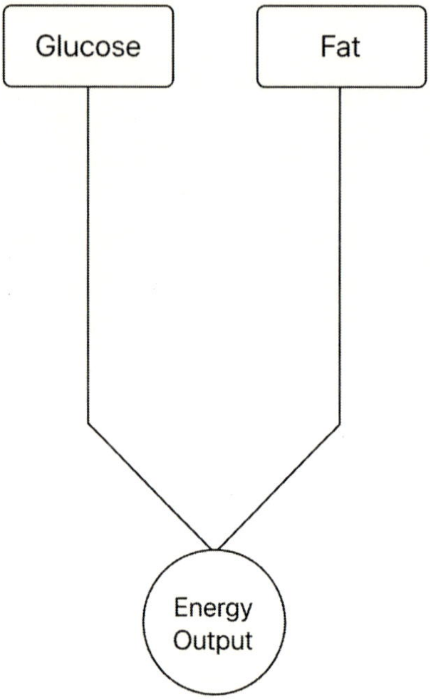

[Figure 1 – Dual Fuel System Map]

This dual availability creates a structural condition in which the system is never dependent on a single source of energy. Instead, it operates through a coordinated balance, where the relative contribution of each substrate shifts in response to internal and external conditions. These shifts are not abrupt substitutions but gradual redistributions, shaped by signaling layers that regulate access, release, and utilization. Insulin, among other signals, plays a central role in modulating this distribution, influencing the degree to which glucose is taken up and the extent to which fat mobilization is constrained. However, the presence of one substrate does not eliminate the other. Both remain within the system, even when one pathway is more active.

The simultaneous existence of glucose and fat as substrates establishes a system that is inherently multi-dimensional. Energy production is not a binary state but a continuum in which both substrates contribute to varying degrees. At any given moment, cells may derive energy from a mixture of glucose and fatty acids, with proportions influenced by factors such as recent input, activity level, hormonal signaling, and overall system state. This mixed utilization reflects the system's capacity to distribute demand across available resources rather than committing exclusively to one pathway.

Availability alone does not determine utilization. The system evaluates conditions that extend beyond simple presence. These conditions include the rate at which substrates can be mobilized, the signaling environment that governs access, and the current demands placed on energy production. Glucose, due to its immediate availability and rapid transport, often contributes significantly when recent input has occurred or when rapid energy is required. Fat, with its larger storage capacity and slower mobilization, becomes more prominent when conditions limit glucose availability or when demand persists beyond immediate input. These distinctions reflect differences in accessibility and response time rather than inherent superiority.

The pathways that process glucose and fat operate concurrently within the system. Glycolysis, glycogenolysis, lipolysis, and beta-oxidation are not mutually exclusive processes. They are regulated in relation to one another, with signaling mechanisms adjusting their activity to maintain coherence in energy supply. This coordination allows the system to adapt to fluctuations without requiring a complete transition from one substrate to another. Instead, adjustments occur through modulation of pathway activity, increasing or decreasing the contribution of each substrate as needed.

Despite this parallel structure, the system does exhibit periods where one substrate becomes dominant in energy production. This dominance is often interpreted as exclusivity, leading to the assumption that the system has shifted entirely to a single fuel. In practice, dominance reflects a relative increase in contribution rather than the elimination of alternative pathways. Even when glucose utilization is elevated, fat metabolism does not cease. Conversely, when fat utilization increases, glucose remains present and continues to contribute, albeit to a lesser extent. The system does not operate through absolute transitions but through proportional adjustments.

This proportionality introduces the concept of conditional exclusivity. Under certain conditions, the system constrains access to one substrate in order to prioritize another. This constraint is not absolute but functionally significant. For example, elevated insulin signaling reduces the rate of fat mobilization, effectively limiting the availability of fatty acids for energy production. At the same time, glucose uptake and utilization increase. The result is a state where glucose becomes the primary contributor, not because fat is absent, but because its access is restricted. The system enforces a degree of exclusivity through constraint, allowing one pathway to dominate while the other remains present but less active.

Conditional exclusivity is governed by the interaction between signaling, substrate availability, and system demand. It reflects a regulatory strategy that prevents conflicting processes from operating at full capacity simultaneously. By modulating access rather than eliminating pathways, the system maintains flexibility while preserving stability. This approach allows for rapid adjustment when conditions change, as the suppressed pathway does not require reactivation from a dormant state but only a release from constraint.

The interpretation of these dynamics often leads to the assumption that one substrate is inherently preferred over the other. Glucose is sometimes described as the body's primary or preferred fuel due to its immediate availability and role in supporting certain tissues. Fat is sometimes framed as a secondary or backup source, engaged only when glucose is insufficient. These interpretations assign qualitative value to substrates based on observed patterns of use, rather than recognizing the underlying conditions that drive those patterns.

Dominance in utilization does not indicate preference. It reflects the alignment of current conditions with the characteristics of a given substrate. When glucose is abundant and signaling supports its uptake, it becomes the dominant contributor because it is readily accessible and efficiently processed under those conditions. When glucose availability is reduced or signaling shifts, fat becomes more prominent because it provides a sustained source of energy that aligns with the system's current constraints. In both cases, the system is responding to conditions, not expressing a preference.

The concept of preference introduces a directional bias that does not exist within the system's regulatory framework. The system does not select substrates based on desirability but adjusts utilization based on availability, signaling, and demand. This adjustment is continuous and responsive, without a fixed endpoint. There is no default state that represents optimal or preferred fuel use. Instead, the system maintains the capacity to distribute energy production across substrates in a way that preserves function under varying conditions.

Misinterpretation arises when snapshots of substrate dominance are treated as defining characteristics of the system. Observing elevated glucose utilization in one context and elevated fat utilization in another can lead to the conclusion that the system transitions between distinct modes with different identities. This perspective overlooks the continuity of underlying pathways and the persistence of both substrates across all states. The system does not adopt a singular identity based on substrate use. It maintains a dual-fuel structure that allows for continuous redistribution rather than discrete switching.

The absence of a preferred fuel is central to understanding the system's organization. Assigning preference implies that one substrate represents a baseline condition to which the system should return or maintain. In reality, baseline conditions are defined by stability, not by the dominance of a particular substrate. Stability emerges from the system's ability to align substrate use with current conditions without accumulating constraint or disrupting coordination. This alignment may involve varying contributions from glucose and fat over time, without privileging one over the other.

The dual-fuel structure provides the foundation for this alignment. By maintaining access to both substrates and regulating their use through coordinated signaling, the system can adapt to changes in input, activity, and internal state. This adaptability does not require a transition from one fuel to another in absolute terms but involves continuous adjustment within a shared framework. The system's capacity to redistribute energy production across substrates is what allows it to maintain function across a range of conditions.

Glucose represents a form of immediate availability within this structure. It is responsive to recent input and can be rapidly mobilized to meet acute demand. Its presence in circulation allows for quick distribution to tissues that require consistent energy supply. Fat represents a form of stored energy, accessible over longer durations and capable of supporting sustained demand when immediate input is limited. The distinction between these roles reflects differences in accessibility and temporal dynamics, not hierarchy.

The integration of these substrates within a single system creates a structure that is inherently flexible. This flexibility is not expressed through constant change but through the capacity to change when conditions require it. The system does not commit to a fixed pattern of substrate use. It maintains the ability to adjust proportions, modulate pathways, and redistribute demand across available resources. This capacity is embedded in the dual-fuel architecture, which allows for variation without requiring reconfiguration of the underlying system.

Understanding this architecture removes the need to interpret energy use through the lens of singular states or preferred fuels. It shifts the focus from identifying which substrate is in use to understanding how the system manages both substrates simultaneously. This perspective emphasizes coordination over selection, continuity over transition, and condition-driven behavior over fixed identity.

The presence of two primary substrates within the system is not a redundancy but a structural requirement. It allows the system to operate across a wide range of conditions without reliance on a single pathway. It provides a buffer against fluctuations in input and demand, enabling the system to maintain function even when one substrate becomes less accessible. This redundancy is not inefficiency but resilience, built into the system's design.

The dual-fuel mechanism establishes the baseline from which more complex behaviors emerge. Without this structure, the system would lack the capacity to redistribute energy production in response to changing conditions. The ability to adjust substrate use is dependent on the presence of multiple pathways that can be modulated independently and in coordination. The system's responsiveness is therefore rooted in its dual-fuel organization.

This organization does not require explicit transitions between fuels to function. It operates through continuous modulation, where changes in signaling and availability shift the balance of utilization. The system remains in a state of dynamic equilibrium, with both substrates contributing to energy production at varying levels. This equilibrium is not static but responsive, maintaining stability through adjustment rather than constancy.

By establishing glucose and fat as parallel substrates within a coordinated system, the dual-fuel mechanism removes the need for hierarchical interpretation. It reframes energy use as a distributed process, where multiple pathways contribute to a shared outcome. This reframing provides a foundation for understanding how the system can adapt to different conditions without relying on fixed states or preferred fuels.

The implications of this structure extend beyond immediate energy production. They define the system's capacity to respond to variability, to maintain function under constraint, and to integrate multiple signals into a coherent output. The dual-fuel mechanism is not a peripheral feature but a central component of metabolic organization. It shapes how the system behaves across time, how it manages resources, and how it preserves stability in the face of changing conditions.

Within this framework, energy use is no longer interpreted as a sequence of discrete states but as a continuous process of allocation. Glucose and fat are not endpoints in this process but contributors, each with characteristics that align with different conditions. The system's behavior emerges from how these contributions are coordinated, not from which substrate is dominant at any given moment.

This coordination establishes the conditions necessary for further mechanisms to operate. The presence of multiple substrates, the ability to regulate their use, and the capacity to adjust their contributions create the environment in which more refined behaviors can occur. The system is structured to accommodate variation, and this structure defines its potential for adaptation.

The dual-fuel mechanism, therefore, is not an isolated concept but the foundational architecture upon which the system's flexibility is built. It defines the range of possible responses by ensuring that multiple pathways remain available and can be engaged in proportion to the system's needs. This architecture does not prescribe outcomes but enables them, providing the structural basis for how the system manages energy across conditions and over time.

Switching Mechanism

The presence of multiple substrates within the metabolic system establishes the conditions under which switching can occur, but it does not, by itself, explain how that switching unfolds. The coexistence of glucose and fat creates the potential for redistribution of energy production, yet potential alone does not define process. Switching emerges from this dual-fuel structure as a regulated sequence of changes that unfold across time, shaped by signaling, availability, and system state. It is not a singular moment in which one substrate is replaced by another, nor is it an instantaneous adjustment triggered by a single variable. It is a coordinated progression in which the relative contribution of each pathway is adjusted through managed transitions.

Interpreting switching as a moment obscures the underlying structure that supports it. A moment implies a discrete shift, a point at which the system moves from one condition to another without intermediate states. In contrast, the metabolic system operates through continuous modulation. The transition from glucose-dominant to fat-dominant energy production involves a sequence of adjustments in pathway activity, substrate accessibility, and regulatory signaling. These adjustments do not occur simultaneously or at identical rates. They unfold with temporal variation, creating a transitional period during which both substrates contribute in changing proportions.

This progression requires that the system alter its internal configuration in a coordinated manner. Pathways that process glucose must reduce their activity while pathways that mobilize and oxidize fat increase their contribution. This change is not achieved by simply activating one pathway while the other becomes inactive by default. It involves active suppression and activation, each governed by signaling mechanisms that regulate enzyme activity, substrate transport, and cellular uptake. The system must manage these opposing adjustments to maintain continuity in energy production, preventing gaps or excesses that would disrupt function.

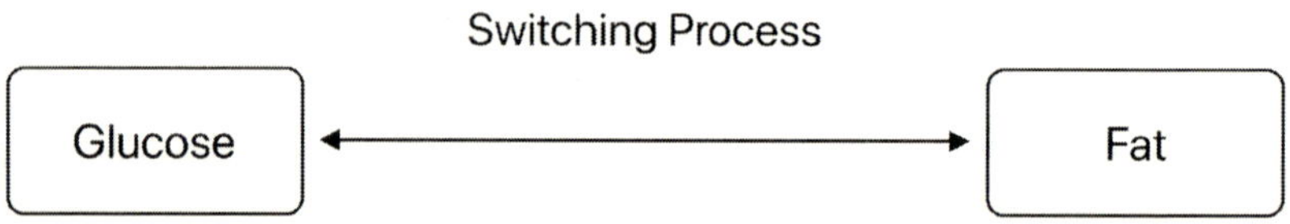

[Figure 2 — Fuel Switching Pathway]

Switching, therefore, is not passive. It does not occur as an automatic consequence of time or absence of input. It requires the alignment of multiple conditions that permit the redistribution of substrate use. These conditions include the signaling environment that governs access to substrates, the availability of those substrates within circulation and storage, and the current demand for energy across tissues. Without alignment, the system cannot transition effectively, even if the underlying pathways are present.

The regulatory nature of switching becomes apparent when examining how pathways are coordinated. Activation of fat utilization requires the mobilization of fatty acids from stored reserves, their transport into circulation, and their uptake into cells where they can be oxidized. At the same time, glucose utilization must be modulated to reflect reduced input or altered signaling. This involves adjustments in insulin signaling, changes in glycogen utilization, and alterations in cellular uptake. These processes are interdependent. Increasing the contribution of one substrate often requires the reduction of the other, not because of mutual exclusivity in structure, but because of regulatory constraints that prevent both pathways from operating at maximal capacity simultaneously.

The system manages this coordination through signaling networks that integrate information about current conditions. Hormonal signals, substrate concentrations, and feedback from tissues contribute to a regulatory environment that determines how pathways are adjusted. This environment does not produce binary outcomes but modulates activity along gradients. As a result, switching is expressed as a gradual redistribution rather than an abrupt change. The system moves through intermediate states where both substrates are active to varying degrees, reflecting the ongoing coordination between activation and suppression.

The initiation of a transition depends on the presence of conditions that allow for reconfiguration of pathway activity. These conditions are not singular triggers but combinations of factors that collectively enable change. A reduction in glucose availability may contribute to the initiation of fat utilization, but this reduction must be accompanied by signaling changes that permit the release and use of fatty acids. Similarly, the presence of stored fat does not ensure its use unless the system's regulatory state allows for its mobilization. Entry into a transition, therefore, is defined by the convergence of availability and permissive signaling.

The completion of a transition is equally dependent on conditions. A shift toward increased fat utilization is not complete when fat pathways are activated; it is complete when the system has reached a new distribution of substrate use that aligns with current conditions. This alignment involves stabilization of pathway activity, where the contributions of glucose and fat reach a balance appropriate for the system's state. Exit from a transition occurs when conditions change again, prompting a redistribution in the opposite direction or toward a different balance. The system remains responsive, with transitions defined by ongoing changes in conditions rather than fixed endpoints.

Entry and exit are not governed by rigid thresholds but by gradients of change. The system does not wait for a specific point to begin or end a transition. Instead, it responds continuously to shifts in availability, signaling, and demand. This continuous response creates variability in how transitions unfold across time. The duration, progression, and intermediate states of switching are shaped by the system's current configuration, which includes factors such as recent input, energy demand, and the integrity of regulatory signaling.

This variability underscores that switching is condition-dependent. The same external circumstance can produce different transitions depending on the internal state of the system. A reduction in input may lead to a gradual increase in fat utilization under one set of conditions and a more constrained adjustment under another. Differences in signaling, substrate availability, and prior system state influence how pathways respond. Switching does not follow a fixed pattern because the system itself is not static. It is continuously shaped by interactions among its components, each contributing to the context in which transitions occur.

The non-uniform nature of switching reflects the system's reliance on coordination rather than predetermined sequences. Each transition is constructed from the current state, incorporating existing levels of pathway activity, substrate distribution, and regulatory signals. This construction process means that switching cannot be generalized as a uniform response. It is specific to the conditions under which it occurs, with variability arising from differences in those conditions. The system does not replicate identical transitions across contexts because the inputs to the process are not identical.

A common interpretation is that the body naturally and automatically switches between fuels as conditions change. This interpretation assumes that the presence of multiple substrates guarantees seamless transitions, independent of system state. It frames switching as an inherent property that requires no coordination, suggesting that the system will adjust without constraint. Such a view overlooks the regulatory requirements that govern pathway activity and the conditions necessary for transitions to proceed.

Switching is not guaranteed. The existence of pathways for both glucose and fat utilization does not ensure that the system can transition between them under all conditions. If signaling does not permit the activation of one pathway or the suppression of another, the transition may be incomplete or constrained. The system's ability to switch depends on its capacity to coordinate these changes, which is influenced by factors such as the current signaling environment and the availability of substrates. Without appropriate conditions, the system may remain in a state where one substrate continues to dominate despite changes that would otherwise favor redistribution.

The assumption of automatic switching also neglects the temporal aspect of the process. Because switching unfolds over time, there are periods during which the system is adjusting but has not reached a new equilibrium. During these periods, substrate contributions are in flux, reflecting ongoing coordination rather than a completed transition. Interpreting these intermediate states as failure or absence of switching misrepresents the process, which is inherently gradual and condition-dependent.

Recognizing switching as a regulated process clarifies its role within the metabolic system. It is not an incidental feature but a core mechanism that allows the system to adapt to changing conditions. By coordinating the activation and suppression of pathways, the system can redistribute energy production in a way that maintains continuity. This coordination ensures that transitions occur without disrupting the overall stability of energy supply, even as the contributions of individual substrates change.

The dual-fuel structure established earlier provides the necessary foundation for this mechanism. Without the coexistence of multiple substrates, there would be no capacity for redistribution. Switching depends on the presence of pathways that can be modulated independently, allowing the system to adjust contributions without requiring complete replacement of one substrate by another. The structure enables the process, but the process itself is defined by how the system manages that structure through regulation.

This management introduces a layer of complexity that extends beyond simple availability. It requires integration of signals that govern pathway activity, coordination of processes that mobilize and utilize substrates, and alignment with the system's current demands. The result is a dynamic process in which transitions are constructed through interaction rather than imposed by a single factor. Switching reflects the system's ability to coordinate its components in response to conditions, maintaining function through controlled redistribution.

The quality of this coordination can vary, influencing how transitions unfold. While the existence of switching is defined by the presence of multiple substrates and regulatory pathways, the characteristics of the transition—such as its progression and stability—are shaped by how effectively the system manages these elements. This variation does not alter the fundamental mechanism but introduces differences in its expression. The system always operates through regulated switching, but the nature of that switching is not uniform.

By framing switching as a process that requires coordination, defined by entry and exit conditions, and shaped by system state, the mechanism becomes distinct from passive interpretations. It is neither automatic nor instantaneous. It is constructed through the interaction of pathways, signals, and substrates, each contributing to the progression of the transition. This construction establishes the basis upon which further properties of switching can be understood, including how transitions differ in their execution.

The system, therefore, is not characterized by fixed fuel states but by its capacity to move between them through regulated processes. Switching is the expression of this capacity, translating the dual-fuel structure into functional adaptability. It exists not as a singular event but as an ongoing process that reflects the system's coordination under changing conditions.

Switching Efficiency Mechanism

Switching efficiency describes the quality of transition across time. The metabolic system may possess the structural capacity to use glucose and fat, and it may contain the regulatory pathways required to move between different patterns of substrate use, but the existence of switching does not determine how well that switching occurs. A transition can be present without being coordinated, complete without being stable, and measurable without being smooth. Efficiency defines the difference between a transition that preserves continuity and a transition that produces disruption as the system redistributes energy production.

Switching, by itself, is not sufficient as an interpretive category. The system is always adjusting substrate contribution in response to input, availability, signaling, and demand. These adjustments occur constantly across gradients, even when the change is too small to be noticed directly. The important question is not whether the system can move between glucose and fat use at all, but how the system behaves while that movement is occurring. A system may eventually increase fat contribution after glucose availability declines, or increase glucose contribution after input rises, yet the period between those states determines much of the functional experience of the transition. The transition itself becomes the site where flexibility is expressed.

Efficiency is defined through speed, smoothness, and stability: speed describes how quickly the transition progresses once conditions permit movement; smoothness describes the absence of abrupt disruption as substrate contribution changes; stability describes continuity of energy supply while the system redistributes activity across pathways. These dimensions operate together because a transition can occur rapidly but unevenly, gradually but steadily, or slowly enough that continuity becomes strained. Efficiency is not identical to speed alone. It is the coordinated relationship between pace, continuity, and system steadiness during the movement from one substrate pattern toward another.

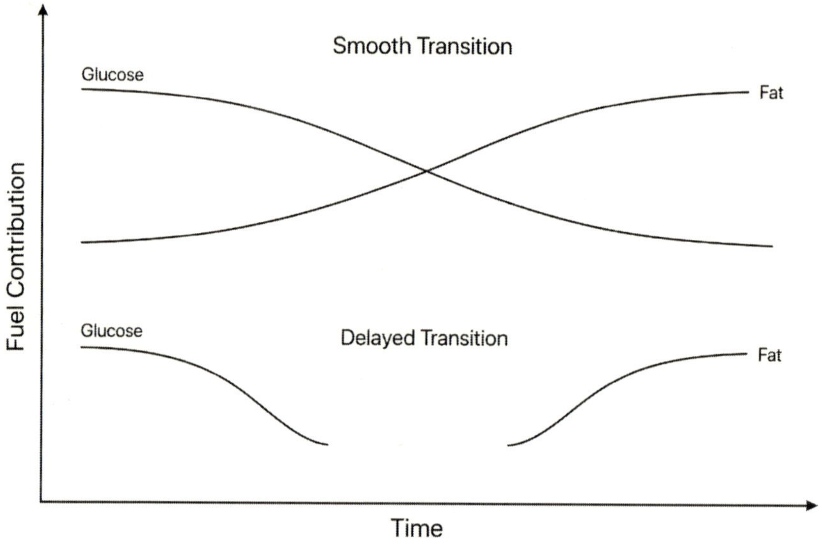

[Figure 3 — Efficient vs Delayed Transition Curves]

The interaction among these dimensions determines whether switching produces coherence or volatility. Speed without smoothness can create abrupt swings in substrate contribution, where pathway activity changes faster than the broader system can integrate. Smoothness without adequate speed may preserve some steadiness but extend the transitional period, leaving the system in an intermediate state for longer than conditions require. Stability depends on both, but it is not merely their sum. It reflects whether energy supply remains coherent while the system changes its internal distribution. A transition can be technically successful while still carrying inefficiency if continuity is disrupted during the process.

The system's ability to transition efficiently depends on its current state. Switching does not begin from a neutral baseline. It begins from the existing configuration of substrate availability, hormonal signaling, tissue demand, glycogen status, and recent input history. A system already operating with coherent signaling and accessible substrate pathways may redistribute energy production with minimal disruption. A system carrying competing signals or constrained substrate access may still switch, but the transition may unfold less cleanly. Efficiency is therefore conditional, not fixed. It is shaped by the state from which the transition begins.

Signaling is central because substrate pathways are not self-directed. The system requires signals that permit one pathway to increase activity while another reduces dominance. Insulin, glucagon, catecholamines, and other regulatory signals influence whether glucose uptake, glycogen release, lipolysis, and fatty acid oxidation are accessible in proportion to current demand. When signaling is coherent, pathway changes can be sequenced in a way that preserves continuity. When signaling is conflicted, the system may receive mixed instructions, producing uneven redistribution. The issue is not simply whether glucose or fat is available, but whether the regulatory environment permits their use in a coordinated manner.

Substrate availability also shapes efficiency. Glucose may be present in circulation, stored as glycogen, or supplied through recent input. Fat may be present in stored reserves but must be mobilized, transported, and oxidized before contributing meaningfully to energy production. These substrates differ in accessibility and timing. Efficient switching requires that availability align with the transition being attempted. When immediate glucose availability declines, the system must increase reliance on stored and circulating fatty acids without allowing energy supply to become discontinuous. When glucose availability rises, the system must accommodate increased uptake while modulating fat contribution. In both directions, efficiency depends on whether the substrate that is becoming more prominent can enter the system at the rate required.

Because switching quality is conditional, it varies across contexts. The same transition can unfold differently depending on prior system state, timing of input, activity demand, sleep disruption, stress load, or accumulated constraint. These conditions alter the signaling environment and the accessibility of substrate pathways. The system may therefore display efficient switching in one context and less efficient switching in another without a change in its basic structure. Flexibility is not a fixed trait expressed identically under all circumstances. It is a capacity whose expression depends on the conditions surrounding the transition.

Delayed transitions occur when the system does not redistribute substrate contribution at the pace required by changing conditions. The pathway that needs to become more active may activate slowly, or the pathway that needs to reduce dominance may remain elevated longer than the new state requires. This delay does not mean switching is absent. It means the transition period is extended. During that extension, the system may operate in a less coherent intermediate state, with demand, availability, and pathway activity not fully aligned. The visible result is not always dramatic, but the internal process reflects reduced efficiency.

Uneven contribution shifts occur when the balance between glucose and fat changes irregularly rather than progressively. One pathway may reduce activity before the other has increased sufficiently, creating a temporary gap in continuity. Alternatively, one pathway may remain dominant while the other begins rising, producing overlap that is not well integrated. These uneven shifts show that switching is not only about movement between fuels, but about proportional coordination during movement. Efficient transition requires the system to adjust contributions in a way that preserves energy flow while changing its substrate mix.

Disruption in continuity becomes most relevant when the system's energy supply feels inconsistent. Energy consistency is often attributed directly to input, as though the presence or absence of food, carbohydrate, or stored energy alone explains the result. Input matters, but it does not operate independently. The system's response to input and absence of input depends on how efficiently it shifts substrate contribution. A system with adequate stored energy can still experience instability if it does not access that energy coherently. A system with recent input can still produce volatility if glucose handling and pathway suppression are poorly coordinated.

Consistent energy reflects smooth transitions more than static fuel use. It does not mean the system remains in one substrate state without change. It means the system changes without creating pronounced interruption. When transitions are efficient, the movement between glucose contribution and fat contribution is absorbed into the broader system without generating instability. The individual may experience this as steadiness, but the mechanism is not subjective motivation or willpower. It is the system's ability to maintain continuity while substrate use is being redistributed.

Volatile energy reflects inefficient transition quality rather than input alone. Rapid rises and declines in perceived energy, uneven steadiness between meals, or pronounced shifts during changing demand can emerge when the system does not coordinate substrate movement smoothly. These expressions are not proof that one fuel is superior or that switching is absent. They indicate that the transition process may be carrying friction. The system is moving, but the movement is not fully coherent. Volatility therefore belongs to the quality of switching, not simply to the identity of the substrate being used.

This distinction matters because metabolic flexibility is often reduced to the ability to use fat or the ability to handle glucose. Those abilities are components, but they do not define the full mechanism. A system may use both substrates and still switch inefficiently between them. It may eventually arrive at the appropriate substrate distribution, yet the transition may be slow, uneven, or destabilizing. Flexibility requires more than access. It requires coordinated movement between states.

The switching mechanism established previously explains how transitions exist. Switching efficiency explains how those transitions are expressed. The first defines the process; the second defines the quality of that process. This distinction prevents metabolic flexibility from being interpreted as a binary capacity. The system is not simply flexible or inflexible. It expresses degrees of flexibility through the efficiency with which it manages transitions across conditions.

Efficiency determines outcome because the transition period is where coordination is tested. A stable endpoint does not erase an unstable transition. The system may ultimately establish a new substrate balance, but the path toward that balance affects continuity. If the transition is delayed, uneven, or disruptive, the system has still switched, but the functional expression of that switch differs from one that occurs with coherence. The quality of movement matters as much as the destination.

Metabolic flexibility, in this framework, is the ability to switch efficiently, not merely the ability to switch. The dual-fuel structure provides the substrate foundation. The switching mechanism provides the regulated process. Switching efficiency defines the system's capacity to preserve speed, smoothness, and stability while that process unfolds. This is the central interpretive lens for understanding flexibility as a stability function rather than a fuel identity. It frames the system not by which substrate dominates, but by how coherently the system moves when dominance changes.

Glucose Utilization Mechanism

Glucose functions within the metabolic system as an externally influenced substrate whose presence reflects both incoming input and internal production. It does not originate as a continuously available resource in the same way as stored energy reserves, but instead enters the system in variable amounts depending on timing, composition of intake, and endogenous regulatory processes such as hepatic glucose release. Once present, glucose is not inert. It represents a signal and a resource that must be actively processed, directed, and integrated into the broader system. Its role is defined not by its presence alone, but by how it is handled once it appears within circulation.

The system treats glucose as a transient substrate that requires immediate regulatory attention. Unlike stored substrates that can remain relatively stable until mobilized, glucose in circulation exists within a constrained range and is subject to continuous adjustment. Its concentration reflects a dynamic balance between entry, removal, and redistribution. Entry occurs through absorption following intake and through internal production mechanisms. Removal occurs through cellular uptake and conversion into other forms. Redistribution involves the allocation of glucose toward immediate use or storage, depending on current conditions. These processes operate simultaneously, creating a continuous flow that must be coordinated to maintain stability.

Glucose does not move directly from entry to use without mediation. Once it enters the bloodstream, it becomes part of a circulating pool that serves as an intermediary stage between input and utilization. This circulating phase allows the system to assess availability and determine how glucose should be distributed. Circulation is therefore not a passive transit stage but an active regulatory domain where concentration, signaling, and demand interact. The system monitors this pool to decide whether glucose should be directed toward immediate energy production or diverted into storage pathways for later use.

Input establishes the initial availability of glucose, but availability alone does not determine its fate. Once present in the bloodstream, glucose must be distributed across tissues that require energy, stored in forms that can be accessed later, or maintained within circulation to preserve stability. This distribution is not uniform. Different tissues have varying capacities for uptake and different roles in overall energy balance. The system must therefore allocate glucose in a way that aligns with both local demand and systemic stability. This allocation is achieved through regulated uptake into cells and controlled storage in specialized tissues.

The pathway through which glucose moves can be understood as a sequence of directed stages. Glucose enters the system through input and internal production, becomes part of the circulating blood glucose pool, and is then allocated through distribution processes that determine its fate. From this distribution point, glucose is directed either toward immediate use, where it contributes directly to ongoing energy demand, or toward storage, where it is converted into glycogen for later access. This sequence—input, circulation, distribution, and allocation—defines the flow of glucose through the system. It is not a linear pathway that proceeds automatically from one stage to the next, but a regulated process in which each stage is influenced by current conditions and system requirements.

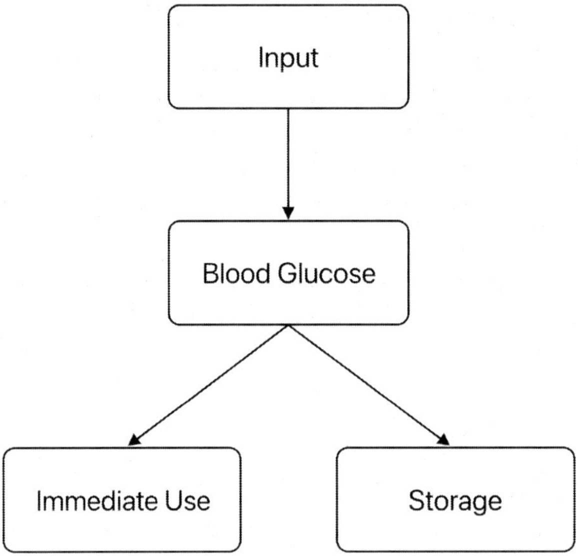

[Figure 4 — Glucose Flow Diagram]

Immediate use represents the portion of glucose that is directed toward active energy demand. Cells that require energy take up glucose from the circulating pool and metabolize it through established pathways to produce usable energy. This process is responsive to demand, increasing when energy requirements rise and decreasing when demand subsides. Immediate use does not imply exclusivity. It reflects the allocation of a portion of available glucose toward current needs, while other portions may be directed elsewhere. The system must balance this allocation to ensure that active tissues receive sufficient substrate without destabilizing the circulating pool.

Storage represents the diversion of glucose into a deferred state, primarily through conversion into glycogen within the liver and skeletal muscle. Glycogen serves as a limited reservoir that can be mobilized when circulating glucose declines or when demand exceeds immediate availability. This storage process is regulated, with capacity constraints that prevent indefinite accumulation. Once glycogen stores approach their limits, additional glucose must be managed through alternative pathways or adjustments in uptake. The existence of storage does not eliminate the need for regulation. It introduces another layer of allocation that must be coordinated with immediate use.

The distinction between immediate use and storage highlights that not all glucose is utilized at the moment it enters the system. Some is directed toward current demand, while some is preserved for future use. This division is not fixed but varies with conditions. When demand is high relative to availability, a greater proportion of glucose may be directed toward immediate use. When availability exceeds immediate demand, a larger portion may be stored. The system continuously adjusts this balance, reflecting the interaction between input, demand, and regulatory signaling.

Glucose utilization is dependent on its availability within the system. Unlike substrates that can be mobilized from large internal reserves, glucose must be present in circulation or generated internally to be used. If circulating glucose declines and internal production does not compensate, its contribution to energy production decreases. This dependency creates a direct link between input and utilization. External input strongly influences how much glucose can contribute at any given time, while internal production provides a secondary mechanism for maintaining availability when input is absent.

This availability dependence distinguishes glucose from substrates that are less constrained by immediate presence. While stored fat can be mobilized over extended periods, glucose requires either recent input or active production to sustain its role. This does not make glucose more or less important within the system, but it does define its behavior. Its contribution fluctuates with availability, and the system must adjust its use accordingly. When availability is high, glucose can play a significant role in energy production. When availability is limited, its contribution decreases, and other substrates must compensate.

Because glucose cannot be used without being present, the system must regulate its availability carefully. Excess accumulation in circulation can disrupt stability, while insufficient availability can limit its contribution to energy production. Regulation therefore operates at multiple levels, controlling entry, distribution, uptake, and storage. These controls ensure that glucose remains within a range that supports both immediate demand and overall system stability. The system does not treat glucose as an unlimited resource but as a variable that must be actively managed.

Insulin functions as a central regulator of glucose distribution within this framework. It does not act as a source of glucose but as a signal that influences how glucose is allocated once it is present. When insulin signaling increases, it promotes uptake of glucose into cells and encourages storage in glycogen. This shifts glucose away from circulation and into tissues, reducing circulating levels while increasing availability within cells. When insulin signaling decreases, uptake is reduced and storage pathways are less active, allowing glucose to remain in circulation or be utilized differently.

The role of insulin is not isolated but integrated into the broader regulatory system. It interacts with other signals that influence glucose production, release, and utilization. Its primary function in this context is to coordinate the distribution of glucose between immediate use and storage. By modulating uptake and storage, insulin helps determine how much glucose is available to different parts of the system at any given time. This coordination ensures that glucose is directed where it is needed while maintaining stability in circulation.

Insulin's influence also extends to how quickly glucose is removed from the bloodstream after entry. Following input, rising glucose levels are accompanied by increased insulin signaling, which accelerates uptake and storage. This reduces the duration of elevated circulation and redistributes glucose into tissues. The rate at which this occurs affects how smoothly the system handles incoming glucose. If uptake and storage proceed in a coordinated manner, the transition from elevated to baseline levels is gradual and controlled. If coordination is less precise, fluctuations may be more pronounced.

The interaction between glucose availability and insulin regulation defines how glucose moves through the system. Availability determines the quantity of glucose entering circulation, while insulin influences how that glucose is distributed and removed. Together, they shape the flow of glucose from entry to use or storage. This flow is not fixed but responsive, adjusting to changes in input, demand, and system state. The system must continuously balance these factors to maintain stability.

Glucose utilization, therefore, is not simply the act of using glucose as fuel. It is a process that includes entry, circulation, distribution, uptake, and storage, all regulated to preserve system coherence. Each stage contributes to how glucose behaves within the system. Disruption at any stage can alter the overall flow, affecting both immediate energy production and the availability of stored resources. The system's capacity to manage these stages determines how effectively glucose contributes to stability.

Within the broader context of metabolic flexibility, glucose represents one side of the substrate distribution that the system must manage during transitions. When conditions favor increased glucose use, the system must handle incoming and circulating glucose in a way that maintains continuity. When conditions shift away from glucose dependence, the system must reduce its contribution without creating instability. The quality of these adjustments is influenced by how well glucose is processed at each stage of its flow.

Switching between substrates involves changes in glucose contribution as well as changes in other pathways. Efficient switching requires that glucose utilization be coordinated with these changes. If glucose handling is uneven, delayed, or poorly regulated, the transition toward or away from glucose use may carry disruption. This does not alter the existence of switching, but it affects how smoothly the transition occurs. Glucose utilization, therefore, plays a role in the broader mechanism of switching efficiency by influencing one side of the transition.

The system integrates glucose utilization with its overall regulatory structure, ensuring that flow, distribution, and control align with current conditions. Glucose is not treated as an independent variable but as part of a network of interactions that determine energy availability and stability. Its behavior reflects the combined influence of input, internal production, distribution mechanisms, and regulatory signals. Understanding glucose in this way shifts the focus from isolated measurements to the processes that govern its movement through the system.

By defining glucose as a controlled flow rather than a static resource, the system's approach to energy management becomes clearer. Glucose enters, moves, and is directed according to conditions, with its contribution shaped by availability and regulation. This perspective removes the need to assign fixed roles or values to glucose and instead emphasizes how it functions within a coordinated system. Its importance lies not in its presence alone but in how effectively it is integrated into the ongoing processes that sustain stability.

Fat Utilization Mechanism

Fat exists within the metabolic system as a stored substrate whose contribution depends on access rather than immediate presence. Unlike glucose, which appears within circulation in response to input and internal production, fat is held in reserve within adipose tissue and must be mobilized before it can participate in energy production. Its presence in the body does not equate to its availability for use. The system maintains large quantities of stored fat, but these reserves are not continuously accessible. Access is controlled through regulatory processes that determine when stored energy can be released, transported, and utilized. This distinction establishes fat as a resource defined by conditional availability rather than constant circulation.

The system treats fat as a reservoir that requires activation. Storage provides capacity, but capacity alone does not determine contribution. Before fat can support energy demand, it must be converted from a stored form into a circulating substrate that can enter metabolic pathways. This conversion introduces structural requirements that differ from those governing glucose. Fat must be released from storage, carried through the bloodstream, taken up into cells, and processed through pathways that allow it to generate usable energy. Each stage introduces a point of control, making fat utilization dependent on coordinated progression rather than immediate response.

The pathway through which fat becomes usable follows a defined sequence. Stored fat is first mobilized through lipolysis, a process that breaks down triglycerides into fatty acids and glycerol. These released fatty acids enter circulation, where they are transported to tissues capable of utilizing them. Once in circulation, they must be taken up into cells, where they undergo further processing to enter energy-producing pathways. This sequence—storage, release, circulation, uptake, and utilization—defines how fat moves from a passive reserve into an active contributor. It is not a direct or instantaneous pathway, but a regulated progression that requires multiple stages to be completed before fat can support energy demand.

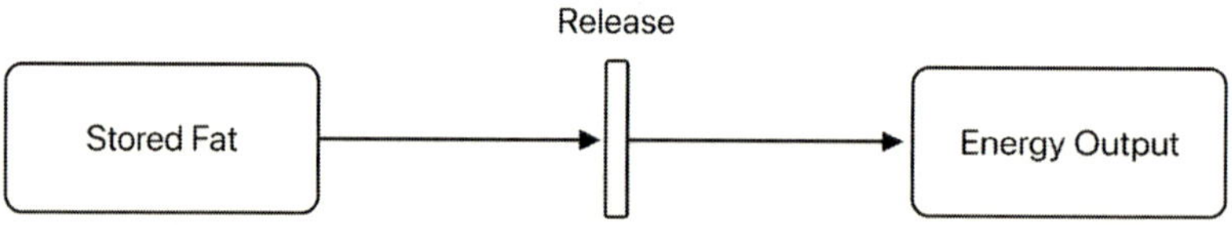

[Figure 5 — Fat Access Pathway]

Release from storage is not continuous. The system does not maintain a constant outflow of fatty acids from adipose tissue independent of conditions. Instead, release is governed by regulatory signals that determine whether mobilization is permitted or suppressed. When conditions favor the use of stored energy, lipolysis increases, allowing fatty acids to enter circulation. When conditions favor the use of alternative substrates, release is reduced, and stored fat remains largely inaccessible. This regulatory structure ensures that fat is not indiscriminately mobilized but is brought into circulation only when conditions align with its use.

The signals that govern release operate within a broader system of coordination. Hormonal influences, substrate availability, and current energy demand interact to determine whether fat mobilization is appropriate. When signaling supports release, the system allows fatty acids to exit storage and become available for use. When signaling suppresses release, access is restricted even though stored fat remains abundant. This distinction emphasizes that mobilization is not a passive consequence of depletion of other substrates but an active process requiring permissive conditions.

The conditional nature of release means that fat cannot be assumed to contribute to energy production at all times. Even when stored reserves are substantial, the system may limit access if conditions do not support mobilization. This limitation is not an error or inefficiency but a regulatory choice that maintains coordination between pathways. By controlling release, the system prevents simultaneous overactivation of competing substrates and preserves stability within energy distribution.

Once fatty acids are released into circulation, they must still be transported and taken up into cells before contributing to energy production. Circulation serves as an intermediary stage, similar to glucose, but with different dynamics. Fatty acids in circulation reflect the current rate of release and the capacity of tissues to absorb and utilize them. Transport proteins facilitate their movement, and their concentration in the bloodstream fluctuates based on ongoing mobilization and uptake. This stage introduces another layer of control, as circulating levels must align with both supply from storage and demand from tissues.

Cellular uptake represents the point at which circulating fatty acids enter metabolic pathways. Cells capable of utilizing fat must take up these fatty acids and direct them into processes that convert them into usable energy. This requires enzymatic activation and transport into specific cellular compartments where oxidation can occur. The process is structured and sequential, adding further dependency on coordinated function. Fat cannot contribute until it has passed through these stages, reinforcing that its use depends on successful progression through the entire pathway.

The need for multiple stages introduces a delay between the onset of conditions that favor fat use and the point at which fat meaningfully contributes to energy production. This delay is not a malfunction but a structural characteristic of the pathway. Mobilization, transport, and uptake each require time, and their coordination determines how quickly fat becomes available. Compared to glucose, which can appear rapidly in circulation and be taken up quickly, fat requires a longer sequence before contributing. This difference in timing reflects the distinct roles of these substrates within the system.

The delay associated with fat activation is therefore inherent to its structure. It does not indicate inefficiency or failure but the necessity of moving through multiple controlled stages. When conditions change to favor fat utilization, the system must initiate release, allow circulation to increase, and facilitate uptake into cells. Each step must align with the others, and the overall process unfolds over time. The result is that fat contribution often lags behind immediate demand when a transition is required. This lag reflects the time required for access to be established rather than a deficiency in the system.

The presence of this delay also highlights the difference between availability and accessibility. Fat is available in large quantities within storage, but it is not accessible until regulatory conditions permit release and the pathway progresses through its stages. Accessibility depends on both the activation of release and the reduction of factors that suppress mobilization. Without both, fat remains in storage regardless of demand.

Access to fat is influenced not only by signals that promote release but also by signals that suppress it. When glucose is abundant and its utilization is elevated, regulatory signals often limit fat mobilization. This suppression reflects the system's coordination between substrates, preventing both pathways from operating at high levels simultaneously.

For fat to become a significant contributor, this suppression must be reduced. The system must shift from a state where glucose dominates to one where conditions allow fat release and use. This shift requires a change in the signaling environment that governs both pathways.

The concept of transition clearance emerges from this interaction. Before fat can be fully activated as a substrate, the system must clear conditions that inhibit its access. This does not involve eliminating glucose but reducing the dominance of pathways that suppress fat mobilization. As these conditions change, release becomes possible, circulation increases, and uptake into cells can proceed. The transition is therefore not only about activating fat pathways but also about adjusting the broader system to permit that activation.

This requirement for clearance reinforces that fat utilization is not independent. It is linked to the state of other substrates and the signals that regulate their use. The system cannot simply initiate fat mobilization without considering the current balance of substrate use. Coordination requires that one pathway increases while another reduces its influence, creating space for redistribution. This interplay defines how transitions unfold and how fat becomes integrated into energy production.

The dependence on both release and clearance means that fat utilization is inherently conditional. It requires permissive signals to mobilize stored energy and the reduction of opposing signals that restrict access. These conditions must align for the pathway to progress effectively. If release is permitted but suppression remains high, mobilization may be limited. If suppression is reduced but release signals are weak, access may still be insufficient. The system must coordinate both aspects to establish meaningful contribution from fat.

Within the broader system, fat represents a resource that can support sustained energy demand once access is established. Its large storage capacity provides a reservoir that extends beyond immediate input, allowing the system to maintain energy production when external availability is limited. However, this capacity is only useful when the system can access it. The regulatory controls that govern release, circulation, and uptake determine whether stored energy can be translated into usable energy.

The integration of fat utilization with other mechanisms highlights its role within metabolic flexibility. Switching between substrates involves not only reducing glucose contribution but also enabling fat access. Efficient transitions depend on how quickly and smoothly this access is established. Delays in release, constraints in circulation, or limitations in uptake can affect the overall quality of the transition. Fat utilization therefore contributes to the broader dynamics of switching efficiency by influencing one side of the redistribution process.

Contrasting fat with glucose clarifies their complementary roles. Glucose reflects immediate availability influenced by input and internal production, while fat represents stored capacity that requires activation. One is present and must be managed, the other is stored and must be accessed. The system relies on both, using regulatory mechanisms to determine when each contributes. This distinction is structural rather than hierarchical, with each substrate fulfilling a different function within the system.

By defining fat as a regulated, condition-dependent resource, its behavior becomes clearer within the context of energy management. It is not continuously active, nor is it automatically engaged when other substrates decline. Its contribution depends on the alignment of release signals, the reduction of suppression, and the successful progression through its activation pathway. These requirements ensure that fat utilization is integrated into the system's broader coordination rather than operating independently.

Fat utilization, therefore, is not simply the presence of stored energy but the process through which that energy becomes accessible and usable. It involves a sequence of controlled stages that transform a passive reserve into an active substrate. Each stage introduces constraints that shape how and when fat can contribute. The system must manage these constraints to maintain stability while adapting to changing conditions.

Within this framework, fat is neither constant nor absent. It is available in storage but conditionally accessible, entering the system through regulated pathways when circumstances permit. Its role is defined by this conditional access, making it a key component of the system's ability to manage energy across varying conditions. The presence of stored fat provides capacity, but its contribution depends on the system's ability to activate and integrate it into ongoing processes.

Understanding fat utilization as a process of access rather than a static resource aligns it with the broader principles of metabolic stability. The system does not rely on continuous activation of all resources but selectively engages them based on current needs and constraints. Fat, as a stored substrate, exemplifies this approach. Its contribution is determined by regulation, coordination, and timing, reflecting the system's capacity to manage its resources in a structured and responsive manner.

Fuel Priority Mechanism

Fuel use within the metabolic system does not arise from selection in the sense of preference or intent. The system does not evaluate substrates and choose between them based on advantage or desirability. Instead, it operates within a structure defined by constraints, where the relative contribution of glucose and fat is determined by regulatory conditions that shape access, activation, and suppression. Priority, in this context, refers to which substrate dominates energy production at a given time, and this dominance emerges from the interaction of signaling, availability, and pathway regulation rather than any form of deliberate selection. The system expresses dominance as a consequence of constraint, not as a result of preference.

The idea of priority often carries an implicit assumption that one substrate is inherently favored over another. This assumption introduces a hierarchy that does not exist within the system's design. Glucose and fat each occupy defined roles within a shared framework, and their contributions shift as conditions change. The system does not assign value to these substrates; it regulates their use according to the constraints imposed by current state. When one substrate becomes dominant, it is because the regulatory environment supports its use while limiting access to the other. Priority is therefore an emergent property of constraint rather than an intrinsic quality of the substrate itself.

The interaction between glucose and fat becomes most apparent when examining how the presence of one influences the accessibility of the other.

Glucose, when present in sufficient quantity and accompanied by the signaling that promotes its uptake and use, exerts a suppressive effect on fat mobilization. This suppression does not eliminate fat from the system but reduces its accessibility by limiting the processes that release stored fatty acids into circulation. At the same time, when glucose influence declines—either through reduced availability or changes in signaling—the suppression of fat mobilization is reduced, allowing stored fat to be released and contribute more significantly to energy production. These opposing adjustments illustrate how dominance is regulated through suppression and release, with both substrates remaining present but contributing unequally based on current constraints.

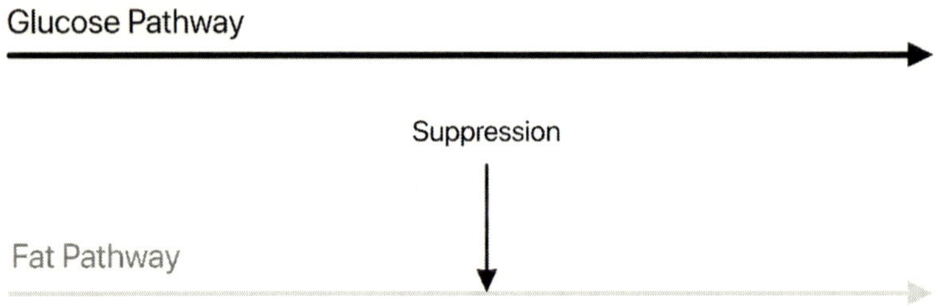

[Figure 6 — Fuel Suppression Model]

Suppression functions as a regulatory mechanism that shapes how substrates interact without removing them from the system. When glucose-related pathways are active and supported by signaling, the system constrains the release of fatty acids from storage. This constraint limits the availability of fat for energy production, even though substantial reserves remain. The system does not require the elimination of fat pathways to establish glucose dominance. It only needs to reduce their accessibility to a level that aligns with current conditions. Conversely, when the factors that sustain glucose dominance diminish, suppression of fat mobilization is relaxed. This allows fatty acids to enter circulation and increases their contribution to energy production. The transition is therefore governed by changes in constraint rather than abrupt substitution.

The regulatory environment determines how these constraints are applied. Hormonal signals, substrate concentrations, and feedback from tissues collectively influence whether pathways are activated or suppressed. Insulin signaling, for example, plays a central role in promoting glucose uptake and limiting fat mobilization, while other signals support the release and use of fatty acids when glucose influence decreases. These signals do not operate in isolation but interact to create a coordinated environment in which substrate use is distributed according to current conditions. The resulting pattern of dominance reflects the balance of these influences rather than any independent action of the substrates.

Constraint-driven priority means that substrate use is an outcome of system state. The system evaluates its internal conditions—such as circulating substrate levels, energy demand, and signaling patterns—and adjusts pathway activity accordingly. This adjustment does not involve a conscious or voluntary process. It is an automatic consequence of regulatory mechanisms that maintain coherence within the system. The pathways that process glucose and fat respond to these mechanisms, increasing or decreasing activity based on the constraints applied. Priority emerges as a result of these responses, not as a directive imposed by the system.

This perspective clarifies that substrate use is not determined by intention. The system does not decide to use glucose or fat based on external directives. Instead, it responds to conditions that influence pathway accessibility. When glucose is abundant and signaling supports its use, the system constrains fat mobilization and establishes glucose dominance. When glucose influence diminishes and conditions permit fat release, the system shifts toward increased fat contribution. These shifts occur because the regulatory environment changes, not because the system chooses one substrate over another.

Dominance patterns are therefore temporary and context-dependent. The system may spend periods in which glucose contributes the majority of energy production, particularly when input is recent and circulating levels are elevated. It may also spend periods in which fat becomes more prominent, especially when glucose availability declines and suppression of fat mobilization is reduced. These patterns are not fixed states but phases within a continuous process of adjustment. The system transitions between them as conditions evolve, with each phase reflecting the current balance of constraints.

The temporary nature of dominance underscores that neither substrate defines a permanent state. Glucose dominance does not represent a baseline condition to which the system must return, nor does fat dominance represent an alternative mode that replaces it. Both are expressions of the same system responding to different conditions. The system maintains the capacity to shift between these patterns, and the transitions are governed by the same regulatory mechanisms that establish dominance. The presence of these patterns reflects the system's responsiveness rather than its commitment to a particular substrate.

Because dominance is driven by constraint, it cannot be directly controlled through isolated actions. The system does not provide a mechanism for selecting substrates independently of the regulatory environment. Attempts to interpret substrate use as a controllable variable often overlook the complexity of the underlying processes. While external factors such as input and activity influence the system, they do so by altering conditions that affect signaling, availability, and pathway activity.

The resulting changes in substrate use are indirect consequences of these influences, not direct outcomes of intentional selection.

This distinction is important for understanding how the system maintains stability. By relying on constraint-driven regulation rather than voluntary control, the system ensures that substrate use aligns with current conditions. This alignment prevents conflicts between pathways and maintains coherence in energy distribution. The system does not require external direction to determine which substrate to use. It integrates information about its state and adjusts accordingly, preserving function through coordinated regulation.

The interaction between glucose and fat also illustrates how suppression and release operate as complementary processes. Suppression reduces the accessibility of one substrate, while release increases the accessibility of another. These processes are not independent but linked through the same regulatory framework. When suppression of fat mobilization is high, release is limited and glucose dominates. When suppression is reduced, release increases and fat contribution rises. The system balances these processes to maintain continuity, ensuring that energy production remains aligned with current conditions.

Within the broader context of metabolic flexibility, fuel priority defines the environment in which switching occurs. Transitions between substrates do not take place in a neutral space but within a system where one pathway is often dominant and the other constrained. Switching involves adjusting this balance, reducing the dominance of one substrate while increasing the accessibility of the other. The efficiency of this adjustment depends on how effectively the system can modify constraints without disrupting continuity.

The quality of switching is therefore influenced by how suppression is managed. If the system reduces suppression gradually and allows release to increase in coordination, the transition can proceed smoothly. If suppression remains elevated while demand shifts, the transition may be delayed, affecting continuity. The interaction between suppression and release shapes how transitions unfold, linking the fuel priority mechanism to the broader dynamics of switching efficiency.

Glucose and fat do not operate as independent fuels that alternate freely. They are components of a coordinated system where the activity of one influences the accessibility of the other. This interaction ensures that the system does not engage both pathways at maximal capacity simultaneously, which could create inefficiencies or conflicts in resource allocation. Instead, it distributes activity according to constraints, allowing one substrate to dominate while the other remains present but less active.

Understanding fuel priority as constraint-driven dominance provides a framework for interpreting substrate use without relying on notions of preference or control. It emphasizes that the system's behavior is governed by regulatory conditions that shape pathway activity. Substrate use reflects these conditions, changing as the system responds to variations in availability, signaling, and demand. The resulting patterns of dominance are temporary, adaptive, and continuously evolving.

This framework integrates the behavior of glucose and fat into a unified system where interaction is central. The system does not treat these substrates as separate entities but as interconnected components whose use is coordinated through constraint. By regulating suppression and release, the system maintains balance between pathways, ensuring that energy production remains aligned with current conditions. This coordination defines how substrates interact and how dominance emerges within the system.

Fuel priority, therefore, is not a directive but an outcome. It reflects the system's response to its internal state, expressed through the relative contribution of glucose and fat. This response is shaped by constraints that regulate access and activity, ensuring that substrate use remains coherent and aligned with demand. The system's ability to manage these constraints determines how effectively it can maintain stability while adapting to changing conditions.

Within this structure, the role of the system is not to choose between fuels but to enforce a distribution that reflects current constraints. This enforcement is continuous, adjusting as conditions change and maintaining alignment between pathways. The system's behavior emerges from this process, with dominance patterns reflecting the balance of suppression and release at any given time. By understanding fuel priority in these terms, the interaction between substrates becomes clearer, and the system's approach to energy management can be interpreted as a coordinated response rather than a series of isolated decisions.

Rigidity Mechanism

Rigidity within the metabolic system emerges when the capacity to switch efficiently between substrates becomes constrained. The system retains the structural components required for switching, and the pathways that support both glucose and fat utilization remain present. However, the quality of transitions deteriorates, and the system's ability to redistribute energy production in response to changing conditions becomes limited. Rigidity does not represent the absence of switching. It reflects a reduction in the system's ability to carry out switching with sufficient coordination, continuity, and responsiveness. The mechanism is defined by diminished flexibility in how substrates are engaged across time.

The reduction in switching capacity alters how the system expresses fuel use. Instead of shifting between substrates in response to variations in availability and demand, the system becomes biased toward one pathway. This bias does not eliminate the alternate pathway but reduces its accessibility and contribution. The dominant substrate maintains a higher level of activity across a broader range of conditions, while the alternate substrate becomes less responsive and more difficult to engage. The result is a pattern in which one pathway remains consistently active, and the other contributes only minimally or under restricted circumstances.

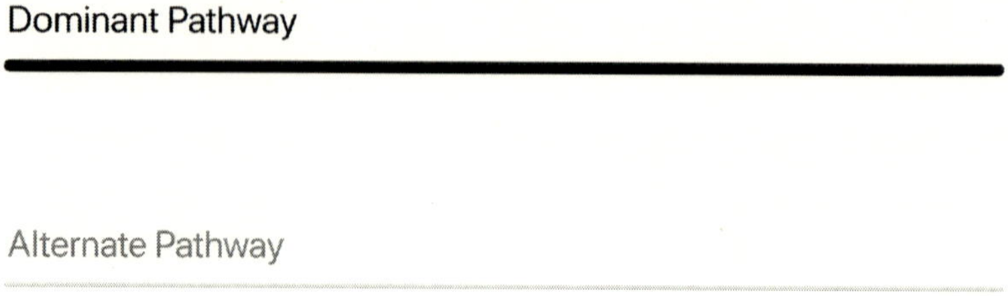

[Figure 7 — Rigid Fuel State Model]

This pattern of dominance represents a form of dependency. The system relies on the dominant pathway to sustain energy production, even when conditions would otherwise support a redistribution. The alternate pathway, while still structurally intact, becomes less integrated into the system's ongoing function. Its activation requires more specific conditions, and its contribution is reduced relative to the dominant substrate. This creates an imbalance in which energy production is concentrated through a narrower set of pathways, limiting the system's ability to adapt.

Limited adaptability becomes evident when the system encounters changes in input, demand, or internal state. Under conditions that would typically prompt a transition, the system's response is slower or incomplete. The dominant pathway continues to carry the majority of the load, while the alternate pathway does not increase its contribution in proportion to the change in conditions. This leads to transitions that are delayed, constrained, or only partially realized. The system still adjusts, but the adjustment lacks the coordination and range that characterize efficient switching.

The reduction in adaptability is not uniform across all conditions. It varies depending on the degree of constraint affecting the alternate pathway. In some contexts, the system may still demonstrate partial switching, with limited engagement of the secondary substrate. In others, the dominant pathway may persist with minimal variation, reflecting a higher degree of rigidity. These differences illustrate that rigidity is not a fixed state but a spectrum defined by how restricted the system's switching capacity has become.

As switching capacity declines, the system's reliance on immediate substrate availability increases. When the dominant pathway is glucose-based, this often manifests as a greater dependence on external input to maintain energy production. Because the alternate pathway—fat utilization—is less accessible, the system has reduced ability to draw on stored resources when glucose availability decreases. This shifts the balance toward a more input-dependent state, where energy stability is more closely tied to the presence of circulating glucose.

This increased reliance on input reflects a narrowing of functional capacity rather than a change in structural components. The system still contains stored energy in the form of fat, but its ability to access and use that energy is constrained. As a result, fluctuations in input have a more direct impact on energy availability. The system's buffer against variability is reduced, making it more sensitive to changes in external conditions. This sensitivity is a consequence of limited access to alternative pathways rather than a deficiency in total energy resources.

Constraint reinforcement contributes to the persistence of rigidity. As one pathway becomes dominant and is used more consistently, the system adapts to support its continued activity. Regulatory patterns, signaling responses, and pathway utilization become aligned with the dominant substrate, making it easier for that pathway to remain active.

At the same time, the alternate pathway, being less frequently engaged, becomes more difficult to activate. This creates a feedback loop in which dominance reinforces itself, further reducing the accessibility of the secondary substrate.

This reinforcement does not require structural change to occur. It operates through adjustments in regulation and pathway responsiveness. The system becomes conditioned to operate within a narrower range of substrate use, and deviations from that range require more substantial changes in conditions. Over time, this leads to a more pronounced imbalance, where the dominant pathway continues to carry the majority of energy production and the alternate pathway remains underutilized.

The persistence of dominance patterns highlights that rigidity is not an abrupt shift but a gradual emergence of constraint. The system transitions from a state of flexible redistribution to one of restricted variability, where switching still occurs but within a limited range. The alternate pathway is not absent, but its contribution is diminished and its activation less consistent. This gradual narrowing reflects the accumulation of constraints that shape how the system responds to conditions.

Within the broader framework of metabolic function, rigidity represents a reduction in adaptability rather than a failure of basic processes. The system continues to regulate substrate use, maintain energy production, and respond to changes in input and demand. However, its responses are constrained by reduced switching capacity, leading to patterns that are less dynamic and more dependent on the dominant pathway. This distinction is important because it frames rigidity as a change in function rather than a loss of function.

The relationship between rigidity and switching efficiency becomes apparent when examining how transitions unfold. Efficient switching involves coordinated changes in pathway activity that preserve continuity and align with current conditions. In a rigid system, these transitions are less coordinated, with delays, incomplete adjustments, or extended periods of dominance. The quality of switching is reduced, even though the underlying mechanism remains present. Rigidity therefore reflects a degradation in the system's ability to execute transitions effectively.

Fuel priority, previously defined as constraint-driven dominance, becomes more persistent under conditions of rigidity. The system continues to establish dominance based on regulatory constraints, but those constraints become less responsive to change. The dominant pathway remains active across a wider range of conditions, and the alternate pathway remains constrained even when conditions begin to shift. This persistence reduces the variability in substrate use, reinforcing the pattern of dependency.

The interaction between glucose and fat under conditions of rigidity illustrates how constraint limits adaptability. When glucose dominance persists, fat mobilization remains suppressed for longer periods, reducing the system's ability to access stored energy. When conditions change to favor fat use, the transition is delayed or incomplete, reflecting the reduced accessibility of the pathway. This interaction demonstrates how rigidity affects both sides of the dual-fuel system, altering not only which substrate is used but how transitions between them occur.

Rigidity also influences how the system responds to fluctuations in demand. Under conditions of increased demand, a flexible system can redistribute substrate use to maintain continuity. A rigid system may rely more heavily on the dominant pathway, even if the alternate pathway could contribute. This reliance can limit the system's ability to adjust efficiently, leading to a narrower range of responses. The system remains functional, but its capacity to adapt is reduced.

The concept of reduced capacity is central to understanding rigidity. The system retains its structural components and basic regulatory mechanisms, but its ability to utilize those components effectively is constrained. This constraint limits the range of conditions under which the system can operate with stability. As a result, the system becomes more dependent on maintaining conditions that support the dominant pathway, rather than adjusting to a wider range of scenarios.

This narrowing of functional range does not imply that the system is static. It continues to respond to changes, but its responses are shaped by the constraints that define its current state. Transitions still occur, but they may require more pronounced changes in conditions to initiate and may proceed with less coordination once initiated. The system's behavior reflects its limited capacity to adjust rather than an inability to adjust entirely.

Within the overall structure of metabolic flexibility, rigidity represents the inverse of efficient switching. Where flexibility allows for smooth, coordinated transitions that maintain stability, rigidity constrains those transitions, leading to patterns that are more fixed and less responsive. The system's ability to manage energy across varying conditions is reduced, and its reliance on specific pathways increases. This shift does not eliminate function but redefines how function is expressed.

Understanding rigidity as a mechanism provides a framework for interpreting changes in substrate use without attributing them to external factors alone. It emphasizes that the system's behavior is shaped by internal constraints that influence how pathways are accessed and coordinated. These constraints determine the system's capacity to adapt, shaping patterns of dominance, dependency, and responsiveness.

By framing rigidity in terms of reduced switching capacity, dominant pathway dependency, limited adaptability, and increased reliance on input, the mechanism becomes integrated into the broader system. It connects the structural components established in earlier chapters with the functional limitations that emerge under constraint. This integration clarifies how the system transitions from flexible to restricted behavior, maintaining continuity while operating within a narrower range of possibilities.

Rigidity, therefore, is not defined by the absence of switching but by the narrowing of its expression. The system continues to function, but its ability to redistribute substrate use is constrained. This constraint shapes how energy is produced, how transitions occur, and how the system responds to change. It represents a shift in capacity, where the system operates with reduced adaptability under the influence of reinforcing constraints.

Transition Delay Mechanism

Transition delay describes a timing misalignment within the switching process, where the system is actively redistributing substrate use but does so with a lag between stages. The transition itself is not absent. Pathways remain functional, and the system continues to adjust its internal configuration in response to changing conditions. However, the coordination between decline and activation is disrupted. One substrate begins to decrease in contribution before the alternate substrate has reached sufficient accessibility to compensate. The result is a temporal gap within the transition, defined not by a lack of total energy resources but by the delay in making those resources available in alignment with demand.

This lag becomes visible when examining how the system manages the handoff between glucose and fat. As glucose contribution declines—whether due to reduced availability, ongoing utilization, or changes in signaling—the system must increase access to fat to maintain continuity. In an aligned transition, this increase occurs in coordination with the decline, allowing one pathway to rise as the other falls. In a delayed transition, this coordination is incomplete. Glucose contribution diminishes while fat access has not yet increased to the level required to sustain supply, creating a gap between ongoing demand and available substrate contribution. The system enters an intermediate state in which both pathways are active but neither is sufficiently aligned with current demand.

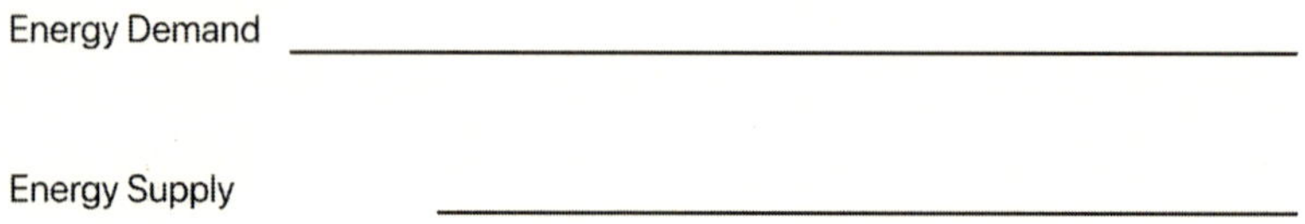

[Figure 8 — Transition Gap Timeline]

This intermediate state reflects a breakdown in timing rather than a breakdown in structure. The system still contains both substrates and the pathways required to use them. The issue lies in the sequencing of activation and suppression. The decline of one pathway proceeds at a different rate than the activation of the other, producing a period where total available contribution does not match the system's continuous demand. This mismatch is transient, but its duration and magnitude define the extent of the delay.

Demand within the system is continuous. Energy requirements do not pause while transitions occur. Cellular processes, maintenance functions, and activity-driven demands persist regardless of how substrates are being redistributed. Supply, however, becomes temporarily misaligned during delayed transitions. The system's ability to meet demand depends on how quickly it can align substrate contribution with ongoing requirements. When timing is coordinated, supply adjusts in parallel with demand.

When timing is delayed, supply lags behind, creating a discrepancy between what is required and what is immediately accessible.

This discrepancy does not indicate that the system lacks energy resources. Stored fat remains available in large quantities, and glucose may still be present at reduced levels. The issue is not absence but accessibility. Fat must be mobilized, transported, and taken up before it can contribute, and this process unfolds over time. When glucose declines more rapidly than fat access increases, the system experiences a temporary gap in effective supply. Energy exists within the system, but it is not accessible at the moment it is needed to maintain alignment.

The structural nature of these gaps becomes clearer when considering how they emerge from the interaction of pathways. Glucose pathways can reduce activity relatively quickly as availability changes, particularly when circulating levels decline or uptake continues without replenishment. Fat pathways, by contrast, require activation through mobilization and transport before they can increase contribution. This difference in timing creates the potential for misalignment. If the decline in glucose outpaces the rise in fat access, the system must pass through a phase where neither pathway fully meets demand.

The duration of this phase depends on the degree of delay in activation. In systems with more coordinated transitions, the lag is minimal, and the intermediate state is brief. In systems where activation is slower or suppression of fat mobilization remains elevated, the lag extends, prolonging the period of misalignment. The system eventually resolves this discrepancy as fat access increases and contribution rises, but the timing of this resolution defines the efficiency of the transition.

Transition delay therefore represents a form of inefficiency within the switching process. It does not prevent switching from occurring, but it alters how the transition unfolds. Efficient transitions minimize the duration of intermediate states by aligning the decline of one substrate with the rise of another. Delayed transitions extend these intermediate states, increasing the period during which supply and demand are not fully aligned. This extension reflects a lack of coordination rather than a failure of pathways.

The role of suppression in shaping this delay is central. When glucose-related signaling remains elevated, fat mobilization is constrained, slowing the increase in fat contribution. Even as glucose declines, the conditions required for fat activation may not yet be fully established. This prolongs the lag between pathways, extending the gap between declining supply and rising accessibility. The system must first reduce suppression before fat mobilization can proceed effectively, adding an additional temporal layer to the transition.

Rigidity amplifies this effect by reinforcing constraints that limit pathway responsiveness. In a system with reduced switching capacity, the activation of fat pathways may be slower, and the reduction of suppression may be less responsive to changing conditions. This combination increases the likelihood of delay, as the system requires more time to adjust its internal state before the alternate substrate can contribute meaningfully. The transition still occurs, but the lag between stages becomes more pronounced.

The misalignment between demand and supply during delayed transitions can be understood as a timing issue within a continuous system. Demand remains stable or changes according to activity, while supply fluctuates based on the progression of the transition. When supply lags, the system operates within a temporary imbalance, relying on incomplete contributions from both pathways. This imbalance resolves as the transition progresses, but its presence defines the inefficiency of the process.

Transition delay also illustrates that switching is not defined solely by endpoints. The system's behavior during the movement between states is as significant as the states themselves. A system that reaches a fat-dominant state after glucose declines may still experience inefficiency if the transition period is prolonged and misaligned. The endpoint does not negate the characteristics of the path taken to reach it. Efficiency is therefore determined by how well the system coordinates timing across the transition, not simply by whether the transition is completed.

The concept of a gap within the transition reframes how energy distribution is interpreted. Instead of viewing energy availability as a static condition, it becomes a function of timing and coordination. The system may contain sufficient total energy, but the distribution of that energy across time determines whether it can meet demand continuously. Delays in activation create periods where availability is effectively reduced, even though resources remain present.

This temporal dimension is central to understanding the role of switching efficiency in maintaining stability. Efficient switching ensures that supply aligns with demand across transitions, minimizing disruption. Delayed switching introduces misalignment, extending the period during which the system operates in an intermediate state. The difference lies in how quickly and effectively the system can coordinate the decline and rise of substrate contribution.

Within the broader system, transition delay represents a specific manifestation of reduced switching efficiency. It isolates the timing aspect of the process, showing how lag between pathways affects overall function. This mechanism does not alter the structural presence of substrates or pathways but changes how they interact across time. The result is a system that continues to function but does so with reduced temporal coherence.

The interaction between glucose and fat during delayed transitions highlights the importance of coordination. Glucose decline is often driven by availability and ongoing use, while fat activation depends on the removal of suppression and the initiation of mobilization. These processes must be synchronized to maintain continuity. When they are not, the system experiences a gap that reflects the difference in timing between them. This gap is not a separate state but part of the transition itself, representing a phase where coordination is incomplete.

By defining transition delay as a lag between depletion and access, the mechanism emphasizes that inefficiency arises from timing misalignment rather than absence of resources. The system's capacity to manage transitions depends on how well it can align the activation of pathways with the decline of others. When this alignment is disrupted, the system moves through a period of reduced coherence, reflecting the extended intermediate state.

The persistence of these delays under certain conditions connects this mechanism to earlier concepts of rigidity and fuel priority. Constraint-driven dominance can prolong suppression of alternate pathways, increasing the time required for activation. Reduced switching capacity can slow the overall progression of transitions, extending the lag between stages. These interactions show that transition delay is not isolated but emerges from the combined effects of constraint, suppression, and reduced responsiveness.

Within this framework, transition delay becomes a defining feature of how the system behaves under constrained conditions. It represents the temporal dimension of reduced flexibility, where the system's ability to align supply with demand across transitions is diminished. The system continues to operate, but its timing becomes less precise, leading to extended periods of misalignment.

This understanding integrates transition delay into the broader structure of metabolic function. It clarifies that energy stability depends not only on the presence of substrates but on the timing of their accessibility. By focusing on the lag between depletion and activation, the mechanism highlights the importance of coordination across time, reinforcing that switching is a process defined by both sequence and timing.

Compensation Mechanism

Compensation within the metabolic system emerges as a response to misalignment created by constrained switching and delayed transitions. It represents a form of short-term stabilization in which the system preserves continuity despite inefficiencies in how substrates are being coordinated. The underlying structure of dual-fuel availability remains intact, and the pathways that govern switching continue to operate. However, when timing between pathways becomes misaligned and accessibility is constrained, the system must adjust to maintain ongoing function. Compensation arises from this need, acting as an adaptive process that sustains energy distribution without resolving the underlying limitations that produced the misalignment.

The defining characteristic of compensation is that it maintains output in the presence of constraint. The system does not suspend demand while transitions are incomplete or delayed. Energy requirements persist, and the system must respond in a way that preserves continuity even when ideal coordination is not available. Compensation therefore operates as a stabilizing layer, redistributing reliance toward the most immediately accessible resources to bridge gaps created by delayed activation or suppressed pathways. This process is not corrective in the sense of restoring full flexibility. It is adaptive in the sense of maintaining function under altered conditions.

A stabilization loop forms when delay within the transition process creates a gap between supply and demand. As one substrate declines and the alternate substrate has not yet increased its contribution sufficiently, the system increases reliance on the substrate that remains most accessible. In many cases, this results in greater dependence on glucose availability, as it can be introduced or maintained in circulation more readily than fat can be mobilized and activated. This adjustment temporarily restores alignment between supply and demand, allowing the system to continue operating without interruption. However, the increased reliance on this accessible substrate reinforces the conditions that limit activation of the alternate pathway, sustaining the original constraint even as immediate stability is preserved.

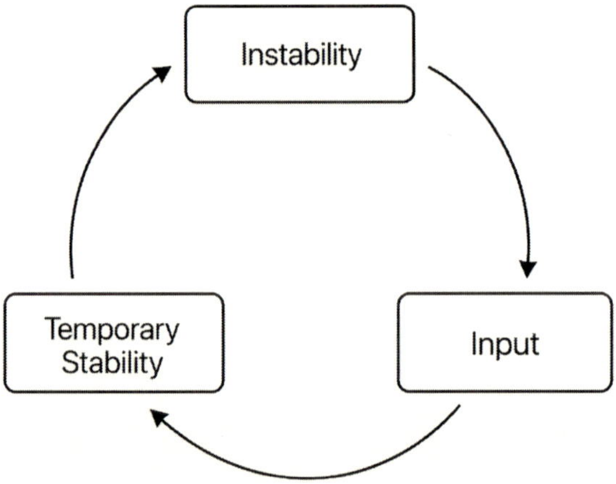

[Figure 9 — Compensation Loop]

This loop structure illustrates how compensation maintains continuity while reinforcing the factors that necessitated it. The system responds to misalignment by amplifying reliance on the pathway that can most quickly restore supply, but this amplification alters the regulatory environment in a way that can prolong suppression of alternate pathways. The system remains stable in the short term, but the conditions required for broader adaptability are not restored. The loop repeats as similar conditions arise, establishing a pattern in which stabilization is achieved through repeated reliance on the same pathway.

Increased reliance on input becomes a central feature of compensation. When the system depends more heavily on substrates that are immediately accessible, external input assumes a greater role in maintaining stability. This does not imply that stored energy is absent or depleted. Rather, it indicates that access to stored pathways is constrained, making internal reserves less available for timely contribution. As a result, the system stabilizes by drawing more consistently from what can be readily introduced into circulation, reinforcing a dependence on availability rather than access.

This shift toward input-based stabilization narrows the system's functional range. Under conditions of efficient switching, the system can balance input with internal resource utilization, distributing reliance across both immediate and stored substrates. Under compensatory conditions, this balance shifts, with input serving as the primary stabilizer and stored pathways contributing less consistently. The system remains functional, but its ability to buffer variability through internal resources is reduced.

The dynamics of compensation also introduce the potential for overcorrection. When the system increases reliance on an accessible substrate to restore alignment, the adjustment may exceed the level required to meet immediate demand. This occurs because regulatory responses are not always precisely matched to the magnitude of the initial misalignment. The system may elevate availability or uptake beyond what is necessary to close the gap, creating a temporary overshoot. This overshoot is not an error but a consequence of operating within a constrained and reactive framework.

Overcorrection produces oscillation around stability rather than stable alignment. The system moves from a state of under-supply relative to demand into a state of over-supply, and then adjusts again as conditions shift. These oscillations reflect the ongoing effort to maintain continuity in the presence of imperfect coordination. The system is not failing to regulate. It is regulating within constraints that limit precision. The result is a pattern of adjustment that maintains function but introduces variability around the target state.

The presence of overcorrection highlights that compensation is not a static adjustment but a dynamic process. The system continually monitors its state and modifies output to maintain alignment with demand. When transitions are delayed or constrained, these modifications become more pronounced, as the system must compensate for gaps that arise during switching. The resulting pattern is one of repeated adjustment, where stabilization is achieved through ongoing recalibration rather than through seamless coordination.

Compensation differs from flexibility in its underlying structure. Flexibility is defined by coordinated transitions that align substrate availability with demand across time, minimizing disruption. Compensation, by contrast, operates when coordination is incomplete. It maintains output by adjusting reliance toward accessible pathways, rather than by resolving the misalignment between pathways. The system remains stable, but the stability is achieved through reactive processes rather than through integrated coordination.

This distinction is critical for understanding the role of compensation within the broader system. Compensation preserves function without restoring the conditions that enable efficient switching. It allows the system to operate under constraint, but it does not expand the system's capacity to adapt to varying conditions. The pathways remain present, and switching continues to occur, but the quality of those transitions remains limited. Compensation addresses the immediate requirement for continuity without altering the structural limitations that define rigidity and delay.

The interaction between compensation and rigidity further illustrates this relationship. In a system with reduced switching capacity, the range of available responses is narrower, making compensatory adjustments more likely. When alternate pathways are less accessible, the system relies more heavily on the dominant pathway to maintain output. This reliance reinforces the existing dominance pattern, creating a feedback loop in which rigidity and compensation support each other. The system remains stable within this loop, but its adaptability is constrained.

Transition delay also contributes to the emergence of compensation by creating the conditions that require stabilization. When timing between pathways is misaligned, the system must bridge the resulting gap to maintain continuity. Compensation provides this bridge by increasing reliance on accessible substrates and adjusting regulatory responses to sustain output. The delay is not eliminated by compensation, but its effects are mitigated in the short term. The system continues to function, even though the underlying misalignment persists.

The feedback nature of compensation ensures that the system remains responsive to changing conditions, even under constraint. As demand fluctuates and substrate availability changes, the system adjusts its compensatory responses accordingly. These adjustments are governed by the same regulatory mechanisms that control normal switching, but they operate within a narrower range of conditions. The system maintains coherence by continuously modifying output, rather than by restoring full coordination between pathways.

The reliance on feedback loops also means that compensation is self-reinforcing. Each compensatory adjustment influences the conditions that shape subsequent responses. Increased reliance on a particular substrate alters signaling patterns, which in turn affect pathway accessibility and activation. These changes can make it more likely that the same compensatory response will be required in the future, reinforcing the loop structure. The system remains stable, but the stability is maintained through repeated application of the same adjustment pattern.

Within the broader framework of metabolic function, compensation represents a mode of operation that prioritizes continuity over adaptability. The system ensures that energy supply remains aligned with demand, even when switching efficiency is reduced and transitions are delayed. This prioritization reflects the system's underlying goal of maintaining function, regardless of the constraints it faces. Compensation is therefore not a deviation from normal operation but an extension of the system's regulatory capacity under altered conditions.

The distinction between stability and adaptability becomes more pronounced in this context. Stability refers to the system's ability to maintain continuous output, while adaptability refers to its capacity to adjust substrate use in response to changing conditions. Compensation preserves stability by maintaining output, but it does so at the expense of adaptability, as it reinforces reliance on specific pathways and limits engagement of alternatives. The system remains functional, but its range of responses is reduced.

By framing compensation as a stabilization mechanism, the system's behavior under constraint can be understood without attributing it to failure or deficiency. The system continues to regulate effectively, using available pathways to maintain continuity. The adjustments it makes are appropriate to the conditions it encounters, even if those conditions limit flexibility. Compensation reflects the system's ability to sustain function, not its inability to operate.

The integration of compensation with earlier mechanisms completes the sequence of how the system responds to reduced switching capacity. Rigidity constrains pathway accessibility, transition delay introduces timing misalignment, and compensation stabilizes output within these constraints. Each mechanism builds on the previous, creating a layered understanding of how the system maintains continuity under varying conditions. The result is a system that remains operational but does so through a different pattern of regulation.

Compensation therefore represents stability under constraint. It ensures that energy supply continues despite inefficiencies in switching and misalignment in timing. It operates through feedback loops that adjust reliance on accessible substrates, maintaining output while reinforcing existing constraints. This process does not restore the system's full adaptability, but it preserves its ability to function, illustrating how stability can be maintained even when flexibility is reduced.

Insulin Interaction Mechanism

Insulin functions within the metabolic system as a regulatory signal that governs access to substrates rather than serving as a substrate itself. It does not contribute energy directly, nor does it act as a source of fuel. Its role is to control how available energy is distributed, determining which pathways are active, which are constrained, and how resources are allocated across tissues. By shaping access and directing flow, insulin operates as a control layer that influences system behavior without participating in energy production. Its effect is indirect but decisive, as it defines the conditions under which substrates can be utilized.

The presence of glucose within circulation introduces a need for regulation, as glucose must be distributed, stored, or utilized in a manner that maintains stability. Insulin emerges as a primary signal in this process, coordinating how glucose moves through the system and how it is made available to cells. When insulin signaling increases, it facilitates the uptake of glucose into tissues, directing it away from circulation and into cellular pathways or storage. This action reduces circulating levels while increasing intracellular availability, aligning distribution with current conditions. The system does not rely on passive diffusion of glucose but on controlled uptake governed by signaling.

At the same time, insulin influences the accessibility of fat as a substrate. Elevated insulin signaling suppresses the mobilization of stored fat, limiting the release of fatty acids into circulation. This suppression does not remove fat from the system but reduces its accessibility by constraining the processes required for its activation. The system maintains fat in storage while prioritizing glucose use, establishing a regulatory hierarchy that reflects current conditions. When insulin signaling declines, this suppression is reduced, allowing fat mobilization to increase and fatty acids to become available for use.

This dual action—promotion of glucose uptake and suppression of fat mobilization—defines insulin as a control gate within the system. It determines which pathways are accessible and which are constrained, shaping the distribution of energy production across substrates. Increased insulin promotes glucose use while limiting fat access, and reduced insulin allows fat activation by removing suppression. The system does not switch substrates independently of this control layer. Instead, insulin sets the conditions under which switching can occur by regulating access to each pathway.

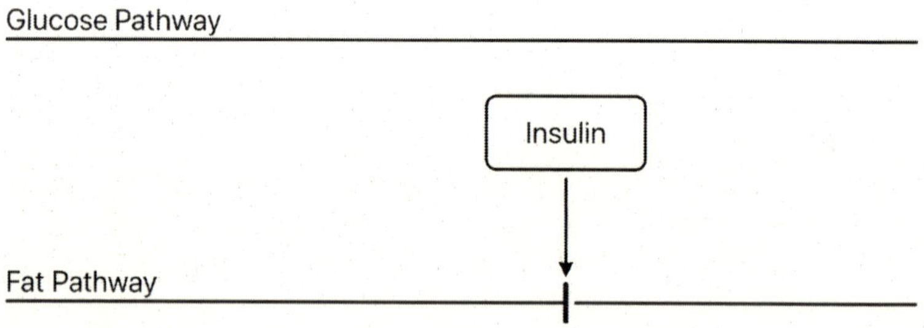

[Figure 10 — Insulin Control Gate]

The regulatory influence of insulin extends to how substrate dominance is established. By promoting glucose uptake and directing it into cells, insulin creates an environment in which glucose becomes the primary contributor to energy production. This effect aligns with the fuel priority mechanism, where dominance is determined by constraint rather than preference. Insulin imposes a constraint on fat mobilization while facilitating glucose use, leading to a state in which glucose dominates because it is both available and accessible. The system responds to this regulatory environment by increasing reliance on glucose pathways.

This enforcement of glucose priority does not imply that glucose is inherently favored as a substrate. It reflects the conditions created by insulin signaling. When insulin levels are elevated, the system is structured to utilize glucose effectively while limiting access to alternative pathways. The resulting dominance is therefore a consequence of regulation rather than intrinsic hierarchy. As insulin signaling changes, the conditions that support this dominance also change, allowing for redistribution of substrate use.

The restriction of fat utilization under elevated insulin conditions illustrates how regulation shapes accessibility. Fat remains present in storage, and the pathways required for its mobilization and use remain intact. However, insulin reduces the rate at which fatty acids are released into circulation, limiting their contribution to energy production. This restriction is not absolute. It operates along a gradient, adjusting the degree of accessibility rather than eliminating it entirely. The system maintains the potential for fat utilization but constrains its expression based on current conditions.

This constraint is central to maintaining coordination between pathways. By limiting simultaneous activation of glucose and fat pathways at high levels, the system avoids conflicting signals and preserves coherence in energy distribution. Insulin's role in this process is to ensure that when glucose is being actively processed, fat mobilization is moderated to match the system's needs. This coordination prevents overextension of multiple pathways and maintains alignment between substrate use and regulatory state.

The influence of insulin on switching timing becomes apparent when considering how transitions between substrates occur. Switching requires that the system reduce reliance on one substrate while increasing access to another. Insulin shapes this process by determining when fat mobilization can begin. When insulin levels remain elevated, suppression of fat access persists, delaying the activation of fat pathways even as glucose availability declines. This creates a lag in the transition, extending the period during which the system operates with reduced alignment between supply and demand.

As insulin signaling decreases, the conditions that restrict fat mobilization are lifted, allowing fatty acids to enter circulation and contribute to energy production. This change marks the initiation of a transition toward increased fat use. The timing of this shift depends on how quickly insulin levels decline and how effectively the system responds to that change. Insulin therefore acts as a temporal regulator, influencing when transitions can begin and how they progress.

The relationship between insulin and transition delay highlights the importance of timing in substrate coordination. Delays in switching are not solely the result of pathway limitations but also of regulatory signals that govern access. When insulin maintains suppression of fat mobilization, the system must wait for conditions to change before the alternate pathway can contribute. This waiting period creates a gap between declining glucose availability and increasing fat access, reflecting a timing misalignment shaped by the control layer.

Compensation mechanisms are also influenced by insulin's regulatory role. When the system encounters a gap between supply and demand, it may increase reliance on accessible substrates to maintain continuity. If insulin signaling supports glucose availability, the system may stabilize by directing more glucose into use, reinforcing its dominance. This adjustment preserves function in the short term but can sustain the conditions that limit fat access, contributing to the persistence of compensatory loops. Insulin therefore participates indirectly in stabilization processes by shaping which substrates remain accessible during periods of misalignment.

The integration of insulin into the broader system reveals its role as a coordinator of interactions rather than an isolated signal. It does not operate independently but in conjunction with other regulatory mechanisms that influence substrate availability and demand. Its primary function is to align distribution with current conditions, ensuring that energy resources are directed appropriately. This alignment involves both enabling access to certain pathways and constraining others, maintaining balance within the system.

By defining insulin as a control gate, the system's behavior becomes more interpretable. Substrate use is not determined solely by availability or storage but by the regulatory environment that governs access. Insulin shapes this environment, influencing which pathways can contribute at any given time. Its presence or absence alters the balance between glucose and fat, guiding the system through different states of dominance and transition.

This perspective clarifies that insulin does not act as a driver of energy production but as a regulator of how energy production is organized. It influences the flow of substrates through the system, determining whether glucose is directed toward immediate use or storage and whether fat remains constrained or becomes accessible. These decisions are not explicit choices but outcomes of signaling interactions that define the system's state.

Within the context of metabolic flexibility, insulin represents the control layer that integrates multiple mechanisms. It enforces fuel priority by establishing conditions for substrate dominance, influences transition timing by regulating access, and contributes to compensation by shaping which pathways remain available during periods of misalignment. Its role is not to determine outcomes directly but to set the conditions under which outcomes emerge.

The presence of this control layer ensures that substrate use is coordinated rather than independent. Glucose and fat do not operate in isolation but are regulated through signals that integrate their activity into a cohesive system. Insulin is central to this integration, providing a mechanism through which the system can adjust distribution in response to changing conditions. Its influence extends across the processes of availability, access, and timing, linking these elements into a unified regulatory framework.

Understanding insulin in this way shifts its interpretation from a singular variable to a system-level regulator. It is not defined by its magnitude alone but by how it interacts with other components to shape behavior. Its effects are expressed through changes in pathway accessibility and timing, influencing how the system transitions between states and maintains stability.

The integration of insulin with fuel priority, transition delay, and compensation mechanisms completes the control layer of the system. It connects the structural and functional aspects of substrate use, demonstrating how regulation governs interaction and timing. By shaping access and suppression, insulin determines how substrates contribute and how transitions unfold, reinforcing its role as a central coordinator within the metabolic system.

Fasting Interaction Mechanism

Fasting, within the metabolic system, is defined as the removal of external input. It is not an intervention in itself but a condition in which incoming substrate from intake is absent, and the system must operate using internally available resources. Under this condition, the continuous inflow of glucose derived from intake is reduced, altering the composition of available substrates within circulation. The system remains active, and energy demand persists, but the sources that supply this demand shift as the absence of input changes the regulatory environment. This shift does not introduce new mechanisms. It exposes the system's reliance on processes that are always present but not always primary.

When external input is removed, the contribution of glucose derived from intake declines as circulating levels are utilized and not replenished through ingestion. Internal production may continue to support some level of glucose availability, but the dominant influence of intake is no longer present. As this external contribution decreases, the system must increase reliance on stored energy to maintain continuity. Pathways responsible for mobilizing and utilizing internal substrates become the primary sources of energy production, and the system redistributes its activity toward these internal resources in response to the absence of incoming supply.

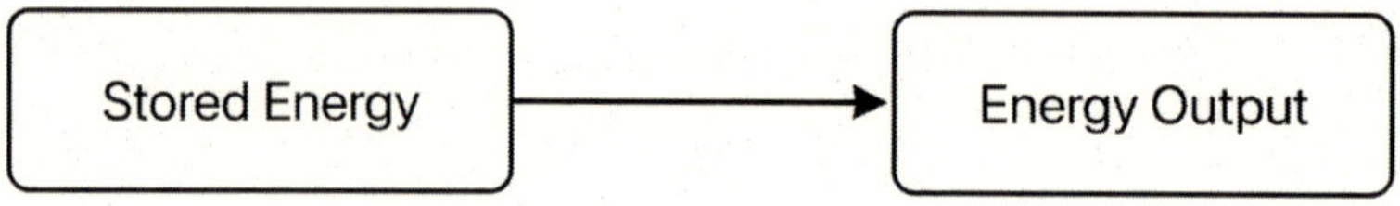

[Figure 11 — Input Absence Model]

This redistribution reflects a shift in dependence rather than a change in structure. The pathways required for internal energy use—particularly those governing fat mobilization and utilization—are always present, but their relative contribution increases when external input is removed. The system does not create new capabilities under this condition. It reallocates existing ones. The absence of input reduces the influence of intake-driven glucose availability and allows internal substrates to assume a greater role in sustaining energy production.

Reliance on internal energy introduces a different set of constraints compared to conditions where input is present. Stored substrates must be accessed, mobilized, and processed before they can contribute. This introduces a dependence on the efficiency of internal pathways and their coordination with ongoing demand. Fat, as a primary stored resource, must be released from storage, transported, and taken up into cells before it can support energy production. The system's ability to maintain continuity under input absence therefore depends on how effectively these processes are activated and integrated.

The transition toward internal reliance is not instantaneous. As external glucose contribution declines, the system must adjust by increasing access to stored substrates. This adjustment unfolds over time, and its progression reflects the system's switching efficiency. In systems where transitions are well coordinated, the increase in internal substrate use aligns closely with the decline in external availability, preserving continuity. In systems where switching capacity is constrained, this alignment may be delayed or incomplete, leading to periods where supply and demand are not fully matched.

Input absence therefore serves as a condition that reveals the characteristics of switching efficiency. Without the buffering effect of continuous intake, the system cannot rely on external supply to stabilize fluctuations. Instead, it must depend on its ability to redistribute energy production internally. The quality of this redistribution—how quickly and smoothly internal pathways are activated—becomes more visible. Efficient systems display coordinated transitions that maintain stability, while constrained systems exhibit delays or extended intermediate states where alignment is reduced.

This exposure does not alter the underlying capacity of the system. It makes existing capacity more apparent by removing an external variable that can mask inefficiencies. When input is present, fluctuations in substrate availability can be offset by incoming resources, allowing the system to maintain stability even if internal coordination is not fully aligned. Under input absence, this external support is removed, and the system's reliance on its internal processes becomes more direct. The result is a clearer expression of how effectively those processes are functioning.

The role of insulin within this context illustrates how input absence modifies the regulatory environment. With reduced external glucose availability, insulin signaling typically declines, decreasing the promotion of glucose uptake and reducing suppression of fat mobilization. This change creates conditions that permit increased access to stored substrates. However, the timing and extent of this shift depend on how the system responds to the absence of input. If insulin remains elevated for a period despite declining glucose availability, suppression of fat mobilization may persist, delaying the transition toward internal reliance.

This interaction between input absence and regulatory signaling highlights the importance of timing in the system's response. The decline in external glucose contribution and the adjustment in insulin signaling must align to facilitate a smooth transition toward internal substrate use. When alignment is present, the system shifts efficiently, maintaining continuity. When alignment is delayed, the system may experience a lag in accessing stored energy, reflecting the same transition delay mechanisms observed under other conditions.

The reliance on internal energy also underscores the distinction between availability and accessibility. Stored substrates are abundant, but their contribution depends on the system's ability to access them in a timely manner. Input absence does not increase the amount of stored energy. It increases the system's dependence on accessing that energy. This dependence brings the processes of mobilization, transport, and uptake into greater prominence, as they determine whether stored resources can be translated into usable energy.

In systems with reduced switching capacity, this dependence can reveal constraints that are less apparent when input is present. If fat mobilization is suppressed or delayed, the system may take longer to establish sufficient internal supply, extending the period of misalignment between demand and available energy. The presence of stored energy does not guarantee immediate contribution. Accessibility must be established through coordinated processes, and any limitation in these processes becomes more visible when external input is absent.

The condition of input absence therefore functions as an exposure layer within the system. It removes the influence of continuous intake and highlights the interaction between internal pathways, regulatory signals, and switching efficiency. The system's behavior under this condition reflects its existing structure and capacity, not a new or altered state. It reveals how the system operates when reliance on internal processes becomes primary.

This distinction is essential for understanding the role of fasting within the broader framework of metabolic flexibility. Fasting does not create flexibility or enhance switching capacity by itself. It does not introduce new pathways or alter the fundamental structure of the system. It places the system in a condition where its existing capabilities are expressed without the moderating effect of external input. The resulting behavior reflects the system's current state, including its strengths and its constraints.

The interpretation of this behavior must therefore remain structural. Variations in how the system responds to input absence are not indicators of intrinsic benefit or harm. They are expressions of how effectively the system can coordinate internal processes under a specific condition. Efficient coordination produces smooth transitions and stable energy distribution, while constrained coordination produces delays or extended intermediate states. These outcomes reflect the system's capacity, not the condition itself.

Within the integrated system, input absence interacts with multiple mechanisms established in earlier chapters. The removal of external input reduces glucose availability, altering fuel priority and shifting dominance toward substrates that can be accessed internally. Insulin signaling adjusts in response, modifying access and suppression dynamics. Switching efficiency determines how well the system transitions between these states, while rigidity and delay influence the presence and duration of misalignment. Compensation mechanisms may emerge if the system requires additional stabilization to maintain continuity.

This integration demonstrates that fasting is not an isolated process but a condition that engages the entire system. It interacts with existing pathways, regulatory signals, and constraints, revealing how they function together when external input is removed. The system's response is therefore a composite of its underlying mechanisms, expressed in the absence of one of its primary variables.

By defining fasting as input absence and examining its effects on substrate availability, regulatory signaling, and switching behavior, the mechanism clarifies its role within the system. It is not a driver of change but a context in which change is observed. The system does not become more or less capable because input is removed. It operates according to its existing capacity, with that capacity becoming more apparent as reliance shifts toward internal processes.

This perspective positions fasting as a diagnostic condition rather than a transformative one. It reveals how the system manages energy when external supply is removed, highlighting the coordination between pathways and the timing of transitions. The behavior observed under this condition reflects the system's current level of adaptability and its ability to maintain stability through internal regulation.

Input absence, therefore, does not define the system's capacity. It exposes it. By removing the influence of external glucose contribution, it brings internal processes to the forefront, allowing the interaction between availability, access, and regulation to become more visible. The resulting patterns are expressions of the system's structure and function, providing insight into how it operates under constraint without altering the underlying mechanisms that define its behavior.

Glucose Interaction Mechanism

Glucose interaction describes the influence of external availability on how the metabolic system organizes substrate use, regulates access, and maintains stability across time. When external input is present, glucose enters circulation in a manner that differs fundamentally from internally derived substrates. Its appearance is not contingent on mobilization from storage but on the direct introduction of substrate into the system. This distinction establishes glucose as a variable whose availability can be continuously reinforced through input, creating conditions that shape how other pathways are engaged or constrained.

The presence of external glucose alters the balance between substrates by changing both availability and the regulatory environment that governs access. Unlike conditions of input absence, where internal pathways must assume primary responsibility for energy production, sustained input presence maintains a consistent contribution from glucose. This consistency reduces variability in substrate availability and stabilizes one side of the dual-fuel system. The system does not interpret this stability as a preference for glucose, but as a reflection of conditions in which one substrate is persistently accessible and therefore able to dominate.

This interaction extends beyond simple supply. Glucose availability influences how the system behaves at a structural level, shaping the conditions under which pathways are activated or suppressed. The system responds not only to the quantity of glucose present but to the regulatory signals that accompany its presence. These signals integrate availability with control, determining how substrates are distributed and how dominance patterns are maintained. Glucose therefore functions as both a resource and a driver of system state, influencing how energy production is organized without acting independently of regulatory mechanisms.

Increased glucose availability leads to an increase in glucose contribution to energy production, supported by signaling that promotes its uptake and distribution. As glucose enters circulation and is maintained through ongoing input, insulin signaling rises in coordination, facilitating the movement of glucose into cells and directing it toward immediate use or storage. This coordinated response ensures that glucose is effectively integrated into the system, aligning its availability with ongoing demand and stabilizing its contribution across time.

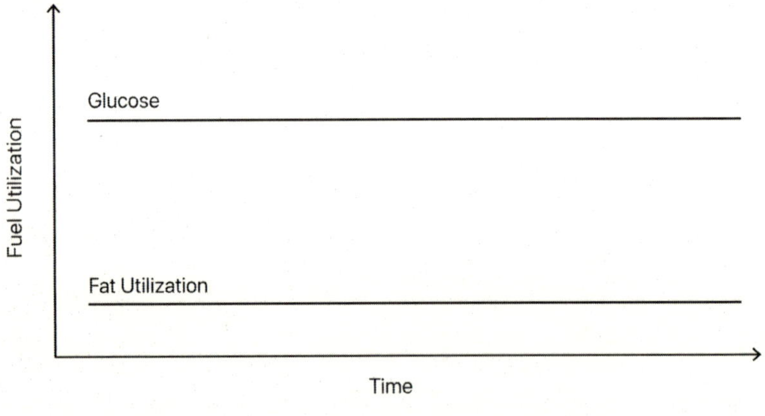

[Figure 12 — Glucose Suppression Curve]

At the same time, insulin-mediated signaling imposes a suppressive effect on fat mobilization. As glucose availability increases and insulin signaling supports its uptake, the release of fatty acids from storage is reduced. This suppression does not eliminate fat from the system but constrains its accessibility by limiting the processes required for its activation. The system maintains fat reserves in a less accessible state while directing energy production toward glucose, creating a condition in which one substrate dominates due to regulatory influence rather than intrinsic hierarchy.

This suppressive interaction emerges from the integration of availability and signaling rather than from the absence of alternate substrates. Fat remains present in storage and continues to exist as a potential energy source, but its contribution is reduced because the conditions required for its mobilization are not met. The system does not deactivate fat pathways entirely. It modulates their activity based on the regulatory environment, allowing glucose to dominate while maintaining the capacity for alternate substrate use if conditions change.

The suppression of fat utilization operates along a gradient rather than as a binary state. As glucose availability increases and insulin signaling remains elevated, fat mobilization is progressively constrained. The degree of suppression reflects the intensity and persistence of the regulatory signals associated with glucose presence. When these signals are sustained, fat access remains limited, and its contribution to energy production is reduced relative to its potential capacity. When signaling diminishes, suppression is gradually lifted, allowing fat mobilization to increase in proportion to changing conditions.

This gradient-based suppression highlights that accessibility, rather than presence, determines substrate contribution. The system may contain substantial fat reserves, but their role in energy production depends on whether they can be mobilized and integrated into metabolic pathways. Under sustained glucose availability, accessibility is constrained, and fat remains a secondary contributor despite its abundance. This distinction reinforces the concept that substrate use is governed by regulation rather than by quantity alone.

The constrained accessibility of fat also influences how the system distributes energy production across time. With glucose consistently available and fat mobilization reduced, the system relies more heavily on a single pathway to meet demand. This reliance simplifies the distribution of energy but reduces the need for coordinated interaction between pathways. The system maintains stability through sustained dominance rather than through dynamic redistribution, reflecting the influence of availability on how substrates are engaged.

Reduced switching demand emerges directly from this condition of sustained availability and suppression. Switching occurs when the system must redistribute energy production in response to changes in substrate availability or demand. When glucose remains continuously available, the system is not required to engage in frequent transitions, as the dominant pathway can meet ongoing energy requirements without adjustment. The need for switching is therefore diminished, not because the system lacks capacity, but because conditions do not require its activation.

This reduction in switching demand affects how often alternate pathways are engaged. When transitions occur less frequently, the system spends more time operating within a stable configuration defined by glucose dominance. Fat pathways remain present but are activated less often, reducing their role in continuous energy production. This dynamic reflects the interaction between availability and pathway engagement, where the presence of a consistent substrate reduces the necessity for redistribution.

The infrequency of switching under sustained glucose availability does not imply that the system loses its ability to transition. The mechanisms required for switching remain intact, and the system retains the capacity to redistribute substrate use when conditions change. However, the expression of this capacity is dependent on variability in input and demand. When variability is low and availability is stable, the system operates within a narrower range of states, reducing the need for transitions and reinforcing the persistence of the dominant pathway.

Switching demand is therefore a function of variability rather than capacity. The system engages in switching when conditions require redistribution, not as a default behavior. When glucose availability remains constant, the system has little reason to shift toward alternate substrates, as the dominant pathway continues to meet demand effectively. This relationship between variability and switching underscores that flexibility is expressed through response to change, not through continuous alternation between substrates.

State persistence arises as a direct consequence of sustained glucose availability and reduced switching demand. Persistence can be defined as the maintenance of a particular substrate dominance over an extended period, driven by stable conditions that reinforce that dominance. When glucose remains available and the regulatory environment supports its use, the system maintains a glucose-dominant state with minimal variation. This persistence reflects the stability of the conditions that define the state rather than an inherent preference within the system.

The maintenance of a persistent state involves the continuation of regulatory signals that support glucose use and suppress alternate pathways. As long as these signals remain active, the system sustains the conditions required for dominance. The result is a stable configuration in which energy production is consistently aligned with glucose availability, and redistribution toward other substrates occurs only when conditions shift significantly. Persistence is therefore a function of ongoing regulation rather than a fixed property of the system.

The extension of this persistent state over time reinforces the interaction between availability and regulation. Continuous glucose availability sustains insulin signaling, which in turn maintains suppression of fat mobilization. This feedback loop preserves the dominant state, ensuring that the system remains aligned with current conditions. The system does not actively maintain this state through intention. It reflects the ongoing presence of the factors that define it, illustrating how stability can emerge from consistent conditions.

Persistence also illustrates how the system balances stability with adaptability. Under conditions of sustained availability, stability is achieved through reduced variability and minimal need for redistribution. Adaptability remains latent, expressed only when conditions change. The system retains its capacity to switch but does not engage it unnecessarily. This balance allows the system to operate efficiently within a stable environment while preserving the ability to respond when variability increases.

The relationship between glucose availability and persistence also interacts with the concept of fuel priority. Fuel priority is determined by constraint, and sustained glucose availability creates a constraint that favors its own use. This constraint is maintained through regulatory signaling, which limits access to alternate pathways and reinforces dominance. As long as the constraint persists, the dominant state is preserved, illustrating how priority and persistence are linked through the same underlying mechanisms.

Integrating this mechanism with earlier chapters clarifies how glucose interaction fits within the broader system. Insulin acts as the mediator that translates glucose availability into regulatory control, shaping access and suppression. The condition of input absence provides a contrast, showing how the system behaves when external availability is removed and internal pathways must assume primary responsibility. Fuel priority explains how dominance emerges under constraint, while switching efficiency determines how transitions occur when conditions change. Glucose interaction ties these elements together by demonstrating how availability influences each layer of the system.

This integration emphasizes that system behavior is not defined by individual variables in isolation but by the interaction between availability, regulation, and constraint. Glucose availability shapes the regulatory environment, which in turn determines pathway accessibility and dominance. The resulting behavior reflects the combined influence of these factors, illustrating how the system organizes energy production under specific conditions.

By defining glucose interaction as the influence of external availability on system state, the mechanism highlights the role of input presence in shaping stability and persistence. It shows that sustained availability can reduce the need for switching, maintain suppression of alternate pathways, and reinforce dominance patterns over time. These effects are not the result of preference or selection but of the conditions created by continuous input and the regulatory responses that accompany it.

The system therefore operates within a framework where availability and regulation determine behavior. Glucose interaction represents one configuration within this framework, characterized by sustained input, reduced variability, and persistent dominance. When conditions change, the system responds by engaging its switching mechanisms, redistributing substrate use to align with new availability patterns. The presence of glucose does not alter the system's capacity for flexibility, but it influences how often that capacity is expressed.

In this way, glucose availability shapes the system's behavior through both direct contribution and indirect regulation. It defines a state in which stability is maintained through persistence rather than through continuous adaptation, illustrating how the system adjusts to the presence of input by aligning its internal processes with external conditions.

Stress Constraint Mechanism

Stress, within the metabolic system, is defined as an increase in system load that alters the conditions under which coordination occurs. This load does not change the structural components that govern substrate use, but it modifies the environment in which those components operate. The pathways responsible for glucose and fat utilization remain present and functional, yet their interaction becomes more complex as load increases. The system must now maintain alignment between supply and demand while operating under heightened signaling pressure, which introduces additional constraints on coordination. Stress therefore functions as a constraint layer, influencing performance by changing operating conditions rather than by altering underlying structure.

The distinction between structure and operating conditions is central to understanding stress within this framework. Structure refers to the fixed components of the system, including pathways, regulatory signals, and substrate availability mechanisms. Operating conditions refer to the dynamic environment in which these components function, including signaling intensity, demand levels, and coordination requirements. Stress modifies these conditions by increasing baseline demand and altering signaling patterns, requiring the system to adjust how it allocates resources. This adjustment does not eliminate existing capabilities but changes how efficiently they can be expressed.

As system load increases, the coordination environment becomes less stable and more variable. Signals that regulate substrate access and distribution must operate within a narrower margin of alignment, and small deviations can have larger effects on overall behavior. The system continues to respond to demand, but the precision of its responses is reduced. This reduction in precision reflects the additional effort required to maintain coherence under load, where multiple processes must be synchronized despite increased variability in signaling and demand.

Cortisol acts as a central regulatory signal within this load state, influencing how the system manages increased demand. Its role is to adjust substrate availability and support energy distribution under conditions that require sustained or elevated response. By increasing internal glucose availability, cortisol ensures that a readily accessible substrate is present to meet immediate requirements. This adjustment modifies the balance between substrates, reinforcing glucose contribution while altering the signaling environment that governs fat access and mobilization. The system integrates this signal as part of its response to load, adjusting its behavior to maintain continuity.

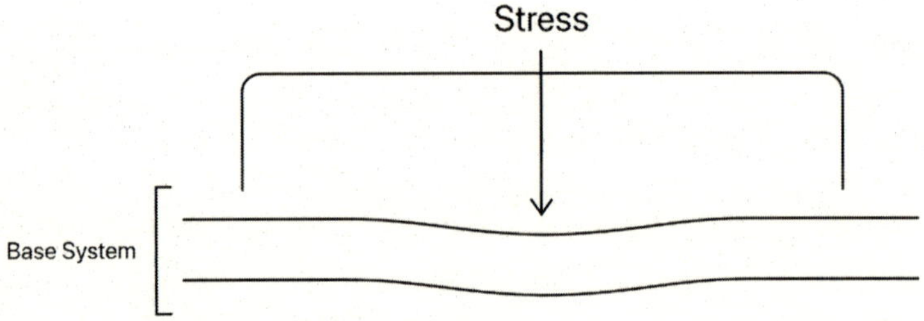

[Figure 13 — Stress Overlay Model]

The influence of cortisol extends beyond substrate availability to the broader signaling environment. It modifies how pathways interact by altering the balance between activation and suppression signals across the system. This creates a condition in which regulatory processes must manage both increased substrate availability and the coordination of multiple signals that may not align perfectly. The system must reconcile these influences to maintain coherence, increasing the complexity of coordination under load. This increased complexity represents an elevation in system demand that goes beyond energy production alone.

Cortisol-driven signaling also raises the baseline level of system activity, requiring the system to operate at a higher level of demand even in the absence of additional external input. This elevated baseline influences how substrates are processed and how transitions occur, as the system must continuously meet higher requirements. The result is a persistent load condition that shapes how pathways are engaged and how efficiently they can coordinate their activity. The system remains functional, but its behavior reflects the additional effort required to sustain operation under these conditions.

Switching between substrates requires coordinated changes in pathway activity, with one pathway decreasing as another increases. This coordination depends on aligned signaling and precise timing, ensuring that transitions occur without disrupting continuity. Under conditions of increased load, the cost of achieving this coordination rises. Cost, in this context, refers to the effort required to align multiple processes, including signaling, substrate availability, and pathway activation. As load increases, the system must expend more effort to achieve the same level of coordination.

The process by which transition cost increases involves multiple steps that unfold across time. Elevated cortisol signaling modifies glucose availability and influences insulin-mediated regulation, altering the balance between substrates. At the same time, the system must respond to increased demand, which accelerates the use of available substrates and shortens the window for coordinated adjustment. These changes create a sequence in which the decline of one substrate and the activation of another are not perfectly synchronized. The system must adjust to these discrepancies, and the effort required to do so represents the increased cost of switching.

Interaction between signaling pathways further contributes to this increased cost. Signals that promote glucose availability may conflict with those required to activate fat mobilization, creating a condition where pathways receive mixed inputs. This conflict slows the process of activation and suppression, as the system must resolve competing signals before transitions can proceed effectively. Timing becomes less precise, and the sequence of events required for smooth switching becomes more fragmented. The system continues to transition, but the process involves greater friction and reduced efficiency.

The consequence of increased transition cost is a reduction in switching efficiency. Transitions become slower, less smooth, and less stable, reflecting the additional effort required to coordinate pathways under load. The system remains capable of switching, but the quality of those transitions is diminished. This diminished quality affects how well the system can maintain continuity, as extended intermediate states and delayed adjustments increase the likelihood of misalignment between supply and demand.

Fuel handling under load reflects the combined influence of altered signaling and increased transition cost. Glucose becomes more consistently available due to cortisol-driven increases in internal production, reinforcing its contribution to energy production. At the same time, fat access becomes less consistent, as mobilization is influenced by competing signals that may not align with current demand. This creates a condition where substrate handling is less predictable and less coordinated, reflecting the complexity of operating under load.

The process of altered fuel handling unfolds through a sequence of interactions between availability, signaling, and pathway activation. Elevated cortisol levels increase glucose availability, while insulin-mediated signals continue to influence uptake and distribution. Fat mobilization is affected by the balance between suppression and activation signals, which may fluctuate as the system responds to changing conditions. These interactions create variability in how substrates are accessed and used, with glucose often dominating due to its consistent availability and fat contributing intermittently based on signaling conditions.

Timing plays a critical role in this process, as the activation of fat pathways may lag behind the system's demand for additional energy. When glucose availability begins to decline or when demand increases beyond its contribution, the system attempts to activate fat mobilization. Under load, this activation may be delayed or inconsistent, reflecting the influence of competing signals and increased transition cost. The result is a sequence where substrate contributions do not align perfectly with demand, creating periods of misalignment.

The consequence of altered fuel handling is a reduction in coordination between availability and use. Substrates may be present but not fully accessible, or accessible but not fully integrated into energy production. This misalignment reflects the system's effort to manage multiple influences under load, where maintaining coherence becomes more challenging. The system continues to function, but its behavior reflects the variability introduced by altered signaling and increased coordination demands.

Stability within the metabolic system is defined as the continuity of energy distribution, where supply aligns with demand across time. Under conditions of increased load, this continuity becomes more difficult to maintain. Stress introduces variability in signaling and increases the cost of coordination, leading to more frequent periods of misalignment. These periods are typically transient, but their frequency and duration increase as load rises, reflecting the system's reduced ability to maintain stable alignment.

The process by which stability is reduced involves a sequence of adjustments that occur as the system responds to load. Increased demand and altered signaling create conditions where substrate contributions fluctuate, requiring the system to adjust more frequently. These adjustments are less precise due to increased transition cost and signaling variability, leading to temporary gaps between supply and demand. The system compensates for these gaps through feedback mechanisms, but the overall continuity of energy distribution is reduced.

Interaction between delay and compensation mechanisms further contributes to reduced stability. Transition delays become more likely under load, as timing misalignment increases and activation of alternate pathways is slowed. Compensation mechanisms respond to these delays by increasing reliance on accessible substrates, often reinforcing glucose dominance. This sequence creates a pattern where stability is maintained through repeated adjustments rather than through coordinated transitions, reflecting the system's effort to operate under constraint.

The consequence of reduced stability is a greater reliance on reactive processes to maintain continuity. The system remains functional, but its operation is characterized by increased variability and more frequent adjustments. This does not indicate a failure of the system but reflects the additional effort required to sustain function under load. Stability is preserved in a functional sense, but its quality is diminished by the variability introduced by stress.

Integrating stress into the broader system framework demonstrates how it amplifies existing constraints without altering structure. Switching efficiency is reduced as transition cost increases, leading to slower and less precise adjustments. Transition delay becomes more pronounced, as timing misalignment is exacerbated by altered signaling and increased demand. Compensation mechanisms become more active, as the system relies on feedback loops to maintain continuity under constraint.

These interactions illustrate that stress functions as a modifier of performance, influencing how effectively the system can coordinate its components. It does not introduce new pathways or remove existing ones, but it changes the conditions under which they operate. The system continues to function, but its behavior reflects the additional load it must manage, leading to reduced stability and increased variability in substrate use.

By defining stress as a constraint layer, its role within the metabolic system becomes clear. It acts as an overlay that increases coordination cost, alters substrate handling, and reduces stability. These effects are integrated with existing mechanisms, shaping how the system responds to increased demand and signaling complexity. The structure of the system remains intact, but its performance is constrained by the conditions imposed by stress, illustrating how load influences the expression of metabolic flexibility.

Electrolyte Constraint Mechanism

Signal transmission integrity within the metabolic system defines the reliability with which information is communicated between pathways that govern substrate use, timing, and coordination. Electrolytes function as the carriers of this information, establishing electrical gradients that allow signals to propagate across cells and tissues. These gradients are not incidental; they are required for the initiation, transmission, and termination of regulatory signals that coordinate metabolic activity. When signal transmission is intact, pathways receive consistent inputs, respond in aligned sequences, and maintain continuity across changing conditions. The system's ability to coordinate transitions therefore depends not only on substrate availability but on the fidelity of the signals that guide their use.

The distinction between fuel and signal layers becomes critical at this point in the system. Fuel represents the material substrate available for energy production, while signal represents the information that determines how that substrate is accessed, distributed, and utilized. Electrolytes operate within the signal layer, enabling communication that organizes fuel use rather than contributing energy directly. This separation clarifies that a system can possess adequate fuel while still experiencing instability if the signaling infrastructure that coordinates its use is degraded. Signal transmission integrity therefore functions as a prerequisite for coordinated metabolic behavior, defining the conditions under which pathways can operate in alignment.

The dependency of coordination on signal integrity introduces a new dimension of constraint. Previous mechanisms have focused on availability, access, and regulation of substrates, but these mechanisms rely on effective communication to function. If signals are not transmitted accurately, the processes that govern switching, activation, and suppression cannot be executed with precision. The system may still attempt to operate, but its behavior becomes less coherent, reflecting inconsistencies in how information is conveyed. Signal transmission integrity thus anchors the coordination layer, ensuring that the system's structural capabilities can be expressed in practice.

Electrolytes act as the coordination layer by enabling the transmission of electrical signals that synchronize activity across metabolic pathways. Their presence supports the generation of gradients that allow cells to respond to regulatory inputs, initiating processes such as substrate uptake, enzyme activation, and pathway modulation. This coordination is not localized but distributed across the system, linking multiple components into a cohesive network. The ability of the system to function as an integrated whole depends on the reliability of these signals, which in turn depends on electrolyte balance.

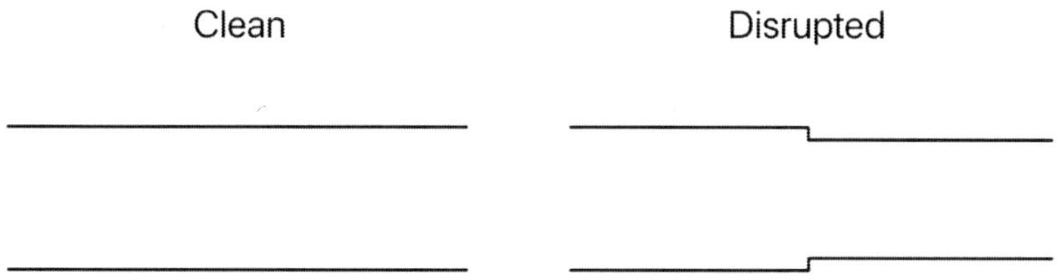

[Figure 14 — Signal Disruption Model]

The role of electrolytes as infrastructure becomes evident when considering how pathways interact. Each process within the metabolic system relies on signals to determine when to activate, when to suppress, and how to adjust in response to changing conditions. Electrolytes facilitate these signals by maintaining the gradients required for their transmission, ensuring that communication occurs with appropriate timing and intensity. When this infrastructure is stable, pathways operate in synchrony, aligning their activity with system demand. The system does not rely on isolated actions but on coordinated sequences of events that depend on consistent signaling.

This coordination layer integrates with substrate use by linking signaling to availability and access. Glucose and fat pathways are regulated not only by their presence but by signals that determine how and when they contribute. Electrolytes enable these signals to reach their targets, ensuring that pathway activation reflects current conditions. The system's ability to transition between substrates, maintain stability, and respond to load is therefore dependent on the integrity of this communication network. Electrolytes, as carriers of this communication, occupy a central role in maintaining coordination across the system.

Disruption within this signaling infrastructure introduces a sequence of effects that alter how transitions occur. When electrolyte balance is compromised, the gradients that support signal transmission become less stable, leading to degradation in how signals are propagated. This degradation affects the initiation of pathway changes, as signals may be delayed, reduced in intensity, or inconsistently transmitted. The sequence begins with impaired signal generation, followed by incomplete or mistimed transmission, and culminates in pathways receiving inputs that do not align with system requirements. The result is a disruption in the coordination required for effective switching.

The timing of this disruption unfolds across multiple stages. Initially, small deviations in signal transmission may produce subtle delays in pathway activation or suppression. As imbalance persists, these delays become more pronounced, leading to extended intermediate states where pathways are neither fully active nor fully suppressed. This creates a temporal mismatch between substrate availability and pathway engagement, similar to transition delay but rooted in signal degradation rather than substrate access. The system attempts to adjust, but the lack of precise signaling prevents it from achieving full alignment.

Interaction between pathways under disrupted signaling further compounds this effect. Signals that should coordinate activation and suppression may arrive out of sequence or with reduced clarity, leading to conflicting instructions across the system. For example, one pathway may receive a signal to activate while another fails to receive the corresponding signal to suppress, resulting in partial engagement of both. This interaction produces a condition where pathways operate without clear coordination, increasing the variability of substrate use. The system continues to function, but the quality of its coordination is diminished by inconsistent communication.

System miscommunication arises when signals fail to align across components, leading to asynchronous behavior between pathways. The process begins with the generation of a regulatory signal that is intended to coordinate multiple processes simultaneously. Under conditions of signal degradation, this message may not be received uniformly, with some components responding while others do not. The result is a breakdown in synchronization, where different parts of the system operate according to incomplete or inconsistent information. This miscommunication disrupts the coherence of metabolic activity, as pathways no longer act in concert.

The timing of miscommunication is characterized by asynchronous responses across the system. One pathway may adjust its activity in response to a signal, while another lags behind or responds with reduced intensity. This creates a sequence in which adjustments are staggered rather than aligned, leading to periods where substrate use does not match demand. The system attempts to reconcile these differences, but the lack of synchronized signaling makes it difficult to achieve consistent alignment. These timing discrepancies contribute to variability in energy distribution, reflecting the impact of signal disruption on coordination.

Interaction between signaling pathways during miscommunication further illustrates how coordination is affected. Insulin signaling, substrate availability, and demand-related signals must align to produce coherent behavior. When electrolyte imbalance disrupts signal transmission, these pathways may operate out of sync, with each responding to different inputs at different times. This interaction produces conflicting patterns of activation and suppression, reducing the system's ability to maintain stable coordination. The result is a state where communication between components is impaired, leading to variability in how energy is managed.

Instability without fuel deficit represents the culmination of disrupted signaling within the system. In this condition, substrates are available, and energy resources are present, but the system cannot coordinate their use effectively. The sequence begins with adequate fuel availability, followed by signal degradation that prevents pathways from accessing or utilizing that fuel in a timely manner. The system attempts to compensate for this lack of coordination, but without reliable signaling, these efforts are less effective. The result is instability that arises not from a lack of resources but from an inability to coordinate them.

The timing of this instability reflects the interplay between signal degradation and system demand. As demand persists, the system must continually adjust its use of available substrates. Under conditions of impaired signaling, these adjustments are delayed or inconsistent, leading to periods where supply does not align with demand. The system may briefly restore alignment through compensatory mechanisms, but without stable signaling, these corrections are not sustained. The instability therefore manifests as repeated fluctuations in energy distribution, reflecting ongoing attempts to coordinate under constraint.

Interaction between compensation and signal disruption highlights the system's response to this instability. Compensation mechanisms increase reliance on accessible substrates to maintain continuity, but their effectiveness depends on the clarity of signaling. When communication is impaired, these mechanisms operate with reduced precision, reinforcing variability rather than resolving it. The system remains functional, but its behavior reflects the limitations imposed by degraded signal transmission. Instability persists despite the presence of fuel, illustrating that coordination is as critical as availability.

The integration of electrolyte constraint with earlier mechanisms clarifies its role within the system. Switching efficiency depends on precise signaling to coordinate transitions, and disruption in this signaling reduces the quality of those transitions. Transition delay can be amplified by signal degradation, as timing misalignment is compounded by inconsistent communication. Compensation becomes more prominent when coordination fails, as the system relies on reactive adjustments to maintain continuity. Electrolyte imbalance therefore interacts with multiple layers of the system, amplifying existing constraints through its effect on signal integrity.

This mechanism shifts the focus from fuel availability to the infrastructure that enables coordination. It demonstrates that metabolic behavior is not determined solely by the presence or absence of substrates but by the system's ability to communicate effectively. Electrolytes, as carriers of this communication, define the conditions under which coordination can occur. When their balance is disrupted, the system's ability to align pathways is compromised, leading to instability even in the presence of adequate resources.

The role of signal transmission integrity within the broader system underscores the importance of coordination as a defining feature of metabolic flexibility. Flexibility is expressed not only through the availability of multiple substrates but through the ability to transition between them in a coordinated manner. This coordination depends on reliable communication, which is supported by electrolyte balance. When this communication is degraded, the system's capacity for coordinated behavior is reduced, illustrating that flexibility is as much a function of signal integrity as it is of substrate availability.

By defining electrolytes as coordination infrastructure, this mechanism expands the understanding of how metabolic systems operate under constraint. It reveals that instability can arise from disruptions in communication, independent of fuel availability. The system remains structurally intact, but its performance is limited by the integrity of its signaling layer. This perspective integrates electrolyte constraint into the broader framework, showing how it interacts with switching, delay, compensation, and stress to shape system behavior under varying conditions.

Aging Constraint Mechanism

Reduced responsiveness within the metabolic system defines a gradual decline in how quickly and precisely the system reacts to changing conditions. This decline does not reflect the removal of pathways or the absence of regulatory mechanisms, but a change in the speed and sensitivity with which those mechanisms operate. Signals that once produced immediate and well-aligned responses begin to generate delayed and less synchronized adjustments. The system continues to detect inputs and initiate responses, yet the timing between detection and execution becomes extended, altering how effectively coordination can be maintained.

The process underlying reduced responsiveness unfolds through changes in signaling transmission, receptor sensitivity, and downstream activation sequences. When a regulatory signal is generated, its propagation across the system may occur with reduced intensity or increased delay. Cells that receive the signal may require longer to initiate the appropriate response, and the magnitude of that response may be diminished relative to earlier conditions. This creates a sequence in which input, transmission, and output are all preserved, but the intervals between them expand, reducing the system's ability to align adjustments with immediate demand.

The system implication of reduced responsiveness is a baseline shift in reactivity, where adjustments occur later and with less precision. This shift affects all layers of coordination, including substrate access, switching behavior, and feedback regulation. The system remains capable of responding to changes, but its responses are less tightly coupled to the conditions that initiate them. This introduces a persistent lag between state changes and system adjustments, establishing the foundation for slower transitions and increased coordination cost in subsequent mechanisms.

Slowed transition dynamics represent the direct expression of reduced responsiveness within switching behavior. Switching between substrates continues to occur, but the processes that govern activation and suppression unfold over longer intervals. The initial signal that initiates a transition is still generated, but the subsequent steps—pathway activation, suppression of competing pathways, and alignment with demand—proceed more gradually. This elongation of transition phases reflects a system that retains its structural capacity for switching but operates with reduced temporal precision.

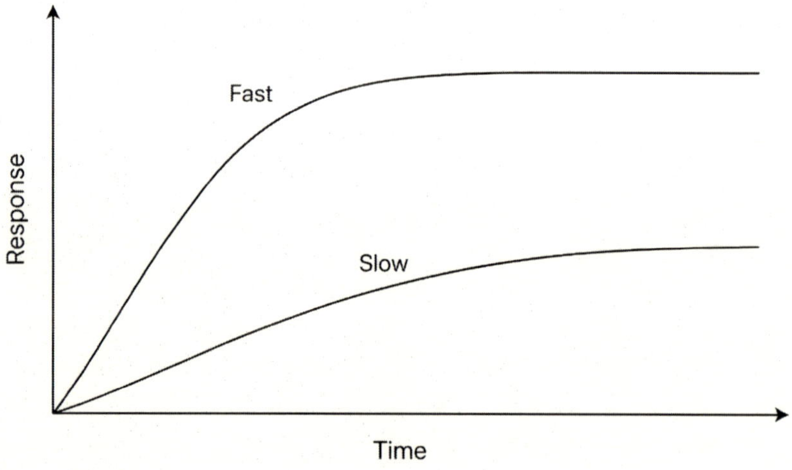

[Figure 15 — Aging Transition Curve]

The sequence of slowed transition dynamics can be traced through each stage of switching. A signal indicating the need for redistribution is generated and transmitted, but the activation of the alternate pathway is delayed relative to the decline of the dominant pathway. Suppression of the initial pathway may persist longer than required, creating overlap between pathways that would otherwise be minimized. The system moves through a prolonged intermediate state, where neither pathway fully aligns with demand. This extended sequence illustrates how reduced responsiveness translates into longer and less coordinated transitions.

Timing plays a central role in this mechanism, as the duration of each transition phase increases under conditions of reduced responsiveness. The interval between signal initiation and pathway activation becomes longer, and the synchronization between pathways becomes less precise. Interaction with other constraints, such as stress and signal integrity, further influences this timing. Under elevated load or degraded signaling, the delays introduced by aging are amplified, creating a compounded effect where transitions become both slower and more variable.

The system implication of slowed transition dynamics is a reduction in switching efficiency, where transitions are less smooth and more resource-intensive. The system must operate within extended intermediate states, increasing the likelihood of misalignment between supply and demand. While switching still occurs, its quality is diminished, affecting the system's ability to maintain continuity under changing conditions.

Accumulation of constraints describes how multiple limitations interact and build over time, shaping system behavior beyond the influence of any single factor. Aging introduces a baseline reduction in responsiveness, but this reduction does not occur in isolation. It interacts with stress-related load, signal integrity challenges, and existing delays in coordination, creating a layered set of constraints that influence how the system operates. Each constraint adds to the overall burden on coordination, increasing the complexity of maintaining alignment between pathways.

The sequence of accumulation unfolds gradually, as repeated exposure to varying conditions reinforces existing limitations. Reduced responsiveness leads to slower transitions, which in turn increase reliance on compensatory mechanisms. Stress introduces additional load, amplifying delays and variability. Signal integrity may fluctuate, further reducing coordination precision. These factors do not act independently; they interact across time, creating a cumulative effect where constraints reinforce one another and become more pronounced.

Timing within this accumulation process reflects the gradual nature of constraint layering. Changes do not occur abruptly but develop over extended periods, with each iteration of system operation contributing to the overall pattern. Interaction between constraints becomes more significant as they accumulate, with stress amplifying the effects of reduced responsiveness and signal degradation further complicating coordination. The system adapts to these conditions, but the cumulative effect is an increase in overall constraint.

The system implication of accumulated constraints is a shift toward operating conditions where coordination requires greater effort and produces less precise outcomes. The system remains functional, but its capacity to manage variability is reduced. Constraints that might be manageable individually become more impactful when combined, leading to a state where coordination is consistently challenged by the interaction of multiple limiting factors.

Progressive rigidity emerges as the long-term outcome of accumulated constraints and reduced responsiveness. Rigidity does not represent the absence of switching but a narrowing of the system's ability to redistribute substrate use effectively. As transitions become slower and less precise, dominance patterns persist for longer durations, and the system becomes less adaptable to changing conditions. This progression reflects a gradual shift from flexible coordination to constrained operation, where the range of possible responses is reduced.

The sequence leading to progressive rigidity begins with reduced responsiveness, which slows transition dynamics and increases reliance on dominant pathways. As transitions become less efficient, the system spends more time in states of prolonged dominance, reinforcing the use of one substrate over another. Compensation mechanisms stabilize these states, further supporting persistence. Over time, this sequence creates a pattern where switching capacity is present but less frequently expressed, and the system operates within a narrower set of conditions.

Timing within progressive rigidity reflects the extension of dominance periods and the reduction in transition frequency. Transitions that once occurred rapidly now take longer to initiate and complete, leading to extended intervals where the system remains in a single state. Interaction with accumulated constraints reinforces this pattern, as stress and signal degradation further limit the system's ability to transition efficiently. The result is a stable but less adaptable system, where changes occur more slowly and with greater effort.

The system implication of progressive rigidity is a reduction in adaptability, where the system becomes more dependent on consistent conditions to maintain stability. This does not indicate a loss of function but a change in how function is expressed. The system continues to operate, but its responses are constrained by the reduced capacity for coordinated transitions, leading to a more persistent and less flexible pattern of substrate use.

Stability under reduced capacity represents the system's ability to maintain continuity despite the presence of multiple constraints. Stability, in this context, is defined as the ongoing alignment between supply and demand, even when the system operates with slower responses and reduced precision. The system adapts to its reduced capacity by narrowing its range of operation, focusing on maintaining consistent output rather than optimizing responsiveness.

The sequence of maintaining stability under reduced capacity involves limiting the extent of adjustments and relying on established patterns of substrate use. Reduced responsiveness leads to slower corrections, and the system compensates by avoiding frequent transitions. This results in a pattern where adjustments are less frequent but more prolonged, allowing the system to maintain continuity within a narrower operational range. Compensation mechanisms play a central role in this process, stabilizing output despite reduced flexibility.

Timing within this mechanism reflects the extension of adjustment intervals and the persistence of intermediate states. Corrections take longer to implement, and misalignment between supply and demand may persist for extended periods before being resolved. Interaction with other constraints, such as stress and signal degradation, further influences this timing, creating variability in how stability is maintained. The system remains functional, but its ability to rapidly restore alignment is diminished.

The system implication of stability under reduced capacity is a form of constrained continuity, where the system maintains function by operating within limits defined by its reduced responsiveness and accumulated constraints. Stability is preserved, but it is achieved through reduced flexibility and increased reliance on consistent conditions. This reflects a system that adapts to its limitations, maintaining coherence through constraint rather than through dynamic responsiveness.

The integration of aging constraint with earlier mechanisms clarifies its role within the broader system. Reduced responsiveness influences switching efficiency by slowing transitions and increasing their cost. Transition delay becomes more pronounced as timing misalignment extends across longer intervals. Compensation mechanisms become more central to maintaining continuity, as the system relies on stabilization loops to offset reduced precision. Stress and signal integrity constraints interact with aging to amplify these effects, creating a system that operates under layered limitations.

This integration demonstrates that aging functions as a time-based constraint on system performance rather than a structural failure. The pathways and regulatory mechanisms remain intact, but their expression is modified by reduced responsiveness and accumulated constraints. The system continues to function, but its behavior reflects a gradual shift toward slower, less precise coordination. This shift defines the long-term trajectory of metabolic flexibility, illustrating how capacity is reduced over time without the loss of fundamental structure.

Continuity Mechanism

Energy flow within the metabolic system is continuous, not segmented into discrete intervals. Demand for energy does not pause between conditions, and the system cannot suspend supply while transitioning between substrates. Instead, it maintains an uninterrupted redistribution of available resources, adjusting contribution levels moment by moment to preserve alignment. This continuity defines the baseline state of metabolism, where energy production is sustained through ongoing adjustment rather than through isolated activation events. The system operates as a flowing process, not as a sequence of separate stages.

The mechanism underlying this continuity is the constant requirement to match supply with demand across time. As energy is consumed, substrates must be mobilized and utilized without interruption, requiring simultaneous engagement of multiple pathways. Glucose and fat are not activated in isolation but contribute in varying proportions depending on current conditions. This proportional adjustment occurs continuously, with no definitive boundary marking the transition from one substrate to another. The system therefore sustains energy flow through overlapping contributions that shift dynamically rather than through discrete changes.

The implication of continuous energy flow is that metabolism cannot be accurately described using segmented models. Any interpretation that divides the system into distinct phases introduces artificial boundaries that do not exist in practice. The system's behavior reflects a continuous redistribution of resources, where each adjustment builds on the previous state. Stability emerges from the ability to maintain this uninterrupted flow, ensuring that energy supply remains aligned with demand even as conditions change.

The absence of discrete modes further clarifies this continuous framework. Terms often used to describe metabolic conditions, such as "fed" and "fasted," do not represent isolated states but points along a gradient of substrate contribution. Glucose and fat are always present within the system, and their relative contributions shift gradually rather than switching abruptly. The system does not enter or exit these conditions in a binary manner; it moves along a spectrum where substrate use is continuously adjusted.

The process by which this gradient operates involves incremental changes in availability, access, and signaling. As external input changes, glucose contribution may increase or decrease, and fat mobilization adjusts in response. These adjustments occur simultaneously, creating a continuum where both substrates contribute to energy production at all times. The system does not disengage one pathway to activate another; it modulates the balance between them. This modulation reflects a continuous process of redistribution rather than a transition between separate modes.

The implication of eliminating discrete modes is that substrate use must be interpreted as overlapping and dynamic. Dominance of one substrate does not imply exclusivity but indicates a relative increase in its contribution within the continuum. The system remains engaged with both substrates, even when one is more prominent. This perspective removes the concept of isolated metabolic states and reinforces the idea that all conditions exist within a continuous spectrum of activity.

Persistent transition state defines the system's ongoing adjustment between substrates. Switching is not an occasional event that occurs only under specific conditions but a constant process embedded within the system's operation. Even when the system appears stable, micro-adjustments are occurring continuously, reflecting small shifts in demand, availability, and signaling. These adjustments ensure that energy flow remains aligned with current requirements.

The mechanism of constant transition can be understood as a sequence without clear boundaries. Each adjustment leads into the next, with no definitive start or end point. Signals that initiate changes in substrate use are continuously generated and acted upon, creating a flow of activity that overlaps across time. This sequence does not resolve into a final state but persists as long as the system is active. Stability within this context is not the absence of transition but the presence of well-coordinated adjustments.

The implication of persistent transition is that the system is always in motion, even when outward conditions appear unchanged. Stability does not represent a static configuration but a condition in which continuous transitions are aligned and balanced. This alignment allows the system to maintain consistent energy distribution while adapting to subtle variations in demand and input. The absence of visible change does not indicate inactivity but reflects the efficiency of ongoing adjustments.

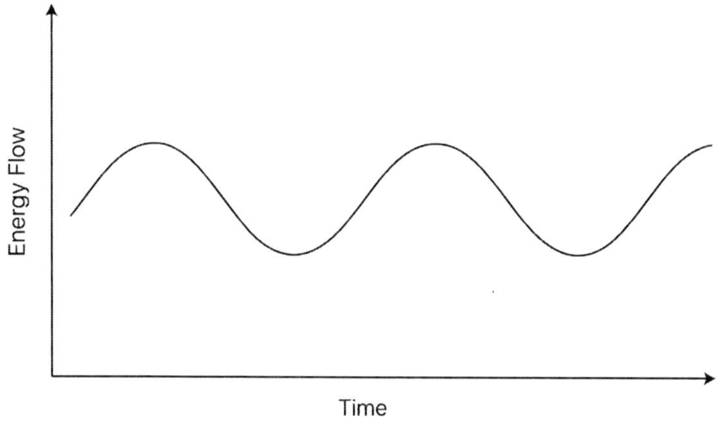

[Figure 16 — Continuous Energy Flow Model]

Overlapping substrate contribution illustrates how glucose and fat coexist within the continuous flow of energy production. Both substrates are active simultaneously, contributing to energy supply in proportions that vary according to conditions. This overlap ensures that the system can maintain continuity even as individual pathway contributions shift. Dominance of one substrate reflects its relative contribution at a given moment, not the exclusion of the other.

The process of overlapping contribution involves coordinated modulation of pathway activity. As glucose availability increases, its contribution rises, while fat contribution may decrease proportionally. When glucose availability declines, fat contribution increases to maintain alignment with demand. These changes occur concurrently, with both substrates remaining engaged throughout the process. The system does not deactivate one pathway to activate another; it adjusts their relative levels of activity within a shared framework.

The implication of overlapping substrates is that metabolic behavior cannot be reduced to single-pathway models. Energy production is distributed across multiple sources, and the system's stability depends on the coordination of these contributions. This overlap provides resilience, allowing the system to adapt to changing conditions without interruption. It reinforces the concept that metabolism operates through integration rather than replacement of pathways.

Stability as continuous alignment reframes the concept of balance within the system. Stability is not defined by a fixed state or the absence of change but by the ongoing alignment between energy supply and demand. This alignment is achieved through continuous adjustment, where small changes in substrate contribution are coordinated to maintain consistency. The system remains stable not because it is static but because its adjustments are synchronized across time.

The mechanism of continuous alignment involves feedback processes that monitor and adjust substrate use in response to changing conditions.

Signals indicating shifts in demand or availability prompt incremental changes in pathway activity, ensuring that supply remains matched to requirements. These adjustments occur rapidly and continuously, preventing large deviations from alignment. Stability is therefore maintained through a series of coordinated micro-adjustments rather than through a fixed configuration.

The implication of defining stability in this way is that change is an inherent feature of stable systems. The absence of change would indicate a lack of responsiveness, not stability. By maintaining continuous alignment, the system preserves consistency in energy distribution while remaining adaptable to variation. Stability is thus a dynamic property, reflecting the quality of coordination rather than the presence of equilibrium.

Instability as flow disruption provides a complementary perspective on system behavior. Instability does not arise from the absence of energy or the presence of incorrect states but from disruptions in the continuity of energy flow. These disruptions can take the form of delays, gaps, or uneven redistribution, where the alignment between supply and demand is temporarily lost. The system may still have adequate resources, but its ability to coordinate their use is impaired.

The process of flow disruption unfolds when transitions between substrates are not properly aligned. Delays in activation or suppression create intermediate states where neither pathway fully meets demand, resulting in temporary mismatches. These mismatches can be amplified by constraints such as stress or signal degradation, which further disrupt coordination. The system attempts to restore alignment, but the presence of disruption introduces variability in energy distribution.

The implication of instability as flow disruption is that it reflects a coordination problem rather than a resource problem. The system's capacity to produce energy remains intact, but its ability to distribute that energy smoothly is compromised. This perspective shifts the focus from availability to coordination, emphasizing that stability depends on the quality of transitions rather than on the presence of substrates alone.

The system is never static, even under conditions that appear stable. Continuous adjustment is required to maintain alignment with changing signals and demand, and this adjustment occurs at all times. Even during periods of rest, regulatory processes are active, modulating substrate use and maintaining energy flow. The system's baseline state is therefore dynamic, characterized by constant activity rather than by equilibrium.

The mechanism of perpetual dynamism involves ongoing interaction between signaling, substrate availability, and demand. Each component influences the others, creating a network of continuous feedback that drives adjustment. This network ensures that the system remains responsive, even in the absence of large external changes. The absence of visible variation does not indicate inactivity but reflects the efficiency of internal coordination.

The implication of a non-static system is that metabolic states cannot be defined as fixed or unchanging. Any apparent stability is the result of continuous regulation, not the absence of movement. This understanding reinforces the concept of metabolism as a dynamic process, where all components are engaged in maintaining alignment across time.

Integration with prior mechanisms reveals how continuity underlies all aspects of system behavior. Switching efficiency determines the smoothness of flow, influencing how well transitions maintain alignment. Transition delay introduces interruptions in flow, creating gaps that disrupt continuity. Compensation mechanisms act to preserve flow when alignment is compromised, reinforcing continuity through reactive adjustments. Stress increases the variability of flow, amplifying disruptions and reducing coordination precision.

Electrolytes contribute to the integrity of signal flow, enabling the communication required for coordinated adjustments. When signal transmission is degraded, the continuity of energy flow is affected, leading to instability even in the presence of adequate resources. Aging introduces a gradual slowing of flow, extending the timing of adjustments and reducing responsiveness. Each of these mechanisms influences continuity, shaping how effectively the system maintains alignment across time.

The integration of these elements demonstrates that all prior mechanisms describe variations in the quality of continuous flow. None of them represent separate behaviors or isolated states; they are expressions of how the system manages ongoing redistribution under different conditions. Continuity provides the framework within which these variations can be understood, linking them into a cohesive interpretation of metabolic behavior.

The metabolic system is therefore always in motion, defined by continuous adjustment rather than by discrete states. Stability emerges from the coordination of this motion, reflecting how effectively the system aligns supply with demand across time. Instability arises when this coordination is disrupted, introducing variability into the flow. By understanding metabolism as a continuous process, the system can be interpreted as an integrated whole, where all components contribute to maintaining alignment within an ever-changing environment.

Context Dependency Mechanism

Identical inputs do not produce identical outcomes within the metabolic system because inputs do not operate in isolation. The system is never encountered in the same configuration twice, and each input interacts with a distinct arrangement of substrate distribution, signaling conditions, and prior transitions. What appears to be inconsistency is a direct consequence of this shifting context, where the same input enters a different system state and therefore participates in a different set of interactions. The variability that follows is not an error in system function but an expression of how the system integrates inputs with its current configuration.

The process by which identical inputs yield different outcomes begins with the point of entry into the system. An input is introduced into an environment defined by existing gradients, active pathways, and ongoing regulatory signals. These factors determine how the input is distributed, which pathways are engaged, and how quickly responses unfold. Even small differences in state—such as slightly altered signaling levels or residual effects from prior transitions—change how the input is processed. The outcome emerges from this interaction, not from the input alone.

The system implication of this interaction is that outcomes cannot be predicted solely by examining the input. Any attempt to establish a fixed relationship between input and response ignores the variability introduced by system state. The same input may contribute to different distributions of substrate use, different timing of transitions, and different patterns of coordination depending on the conditions under which it is introduced. This establishes variability as a structural feature of the system, rooted in context rather than randomness.

System state functions as the controlling variable that shapes how inputs are processed and how responses are expressed. This state is defined by multiple overlapping factors, including current substrate distribution, prevailing signaling conditions, recent transition history, and the presence of constraints such as stress or signal degradation. Each of these components contributes to the configuration of the system at a given moment, creating a dynamic environment in which inputs are interpreted and acted upon. The system does not respond to inputs in isolation; it responds according to the configuration in which those inputs are received.

The mechanism of state-dependent response unfolds through the interaction between input and existing conditions. When an input enters the system, it encounters pathways that are already active to varying degrees, signals that are already influencing distribution, and constraints that are already shaping coordination. These factors determine the relative contribution of different substrates, the timing of activation and suppression, and the degree of alignment between supply and demand. The response reflects the interaction between input and state, not a direct translation of input into outcome.

The system implication of state-dependent response is that interpretation must account for the configuration of the system at the time of input. Without this context, the relationship between input and outcome cannot be accurately understood. The same input may amplify an existing pathway in one state, initiate a transition in another, or be integrated with minimal disruption in a third. Each outcome is valid within its context, reinforcing that responses are conditional rather than absolute.

Prior conditions contribute to the formation of system state by carrying the effects of previous inputs, transitions, and constraints forward into the present. The system does not reset between events; it retains the influence of what has occurred previously, integrating these effects into its current configuration. This continuity means that each new input is processed within a context shaped by prior activity, creating a chain of dependency that links past and present conditions. The system's behavior is therefore cumulative, reflecting the integration of its history.

The process of temporal dependency involves the gradual accumulation of changes across time. Previous inputs influence substrate distribution, prior transitions alter pathway engagement, and accumulated constraints modify signaling and coordination. These factors do not dissipate immediately but persist, shaping the conditions under which subsequent inputs are processed. The system carries this history forward, creating a layered context in which each new input participates.

The system implication of prior conditions is that outcomes are influenced by sequences rather than isolated events. A given response cannot be understood without considering the conditions that preceded it, as these conditions determine how the system is configured at the moment of input. This reinforces the concept that metabolic behavior is path-dependent, where the trajectory leading to a given state influences how that state responds to new inputs.

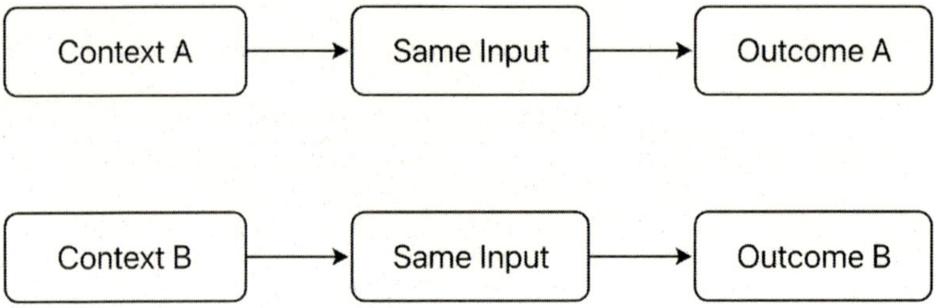

[Figure 17 — Context Split Model]

Temporal layering of state describes how the system builds its configuration over time through the accumulation of prior conditions. Each input, transition, and constraint contributes to the ongoing construction of state, creating a layered structure that evolves continuously. There is no point at which the system returns to a neutral baseline; instead, each condition modifies the existing configuration, adding to its complexity. This layering ensures that the system is always operating within a context shaped by its history.

The process of temporal layering unfolds through the sequential integration of events. An input alters substrate distribution and signaling, which influences subsequent transitions. These transitions modify pathway engagement, which in turn affects how future inputs are processed. Constraints such as stress or signal degradation interact with these changes, further shaping the system's configuration. Over time, these layers accumulate, creating a context that reflects the combined influence of multiple factors.

The system implication of temporal layering is that outcomes depend on sequences rather than moments. A single input cannot be isolated from the conditions that precede and follow it, as these conditions define the context in which it operates. This path dependency ensures that responses are not only state-dependent but also sequence-dependent, reinforcing the importance of temporal context in interpreting system behavior.

Interaction of multiple variables within the system creates outcomes that emerge from the combined influence of inputs, signaling, availability, constraints, and demand. No single variable operates independently; each interacts with others to shape the system's response. Inputs modify substrate availability, signaling influences pathway activation, constraints alter coordination, and demand drives redistribution. The outcome reflects the integration of these factors, not the effect of any one variable in isolation.

The process of multi-variable interaction involves simultaneous adjustments across multiple layers of the system. When an input is introduced, it interacts with existing signaling conditions, which may amplify or suppress its effects. Substrate availability influences how the input is distributed, while constraints modify the timing and coordination of responses. These interactions occur concurrently, creating a network of influences that shape the final outcome. The system's behavior emerges from this network, not from a single causal pathway.

The system implication of multi-variable interaction is that interpretation requires an understanding of how variables combine rather than how they act individually. Simplifying the system to a single cause-and-effect relationship removes the context necessary to understand its behavior. Outcomes are composite results, reflecting the integration of multiple influences that vary across time and conditions.

Failure of isolated interpretation arises when attempts are made to analyze metabolic behavior without accounting for context. Observing a single event and attributing its outcome to a single input ignores the influence of system state, prior conditions, and interacting variables. This approach reduces a complex system to a simplified model that cannot capture its dynamics. As a result, conclusions drawn from isolated analysis are incomplete and often misleading.

The process leading to interpretive failure begins with the assumption that inputs operate independently. This assumption overlooks the role of state and interaction, treating outcomes as direct consequences of inputs rather than as products of context. Without considering the configuration of the system, the timing of events, and the influence of constraints, the analysis lacks the information necessary to accurately interpret behavior. The system's responses appear inconsistent or unpredictable when viewed through this limited lens.

The system implication of this failure is that meaningful interpretation requires integration of context. Observations must be understood as part of a broader sequence, where inputs interact with state and contribute to ongoing processes. Removing context eliminates the conditions that define how the system operates, making it impossible to accurately interpret outcomes.

Variability within the system is structural, reflecting changes in state rather than random fluctuations. As the system continuously adjusts to evolving conditions, its responses naturally vary, producing differences in outcomes even when inputs appear similar. This variability is an expected feature of a system that operates through continuous flow and context-dependent interaction. It indicates that the system is responding to its current configuration, not that it is malfunctioning.

The process by which variability emerges involves the ongoing modification of state through inputs, transitions, and constraints. Each adjustment alters the system's configuration, influencing how subsequent inputs are processed. As these changes accumulate, the system produces a range of responses that reflect its evolving context. This variability is therefore a direct expression of the system's dynamic nature.

The system implication of structural variability is that consistency cannot be defined as identical outcomes under identical inputs. Instead, consistency is reflected in the system's ability to maintain alignment across varying conditions. Variability becomes a measure of context, indicating how the system adapts to changing configurations rather than how it deviates from a fixed pattern.

Integration with continuous flow reinforces the connection between context and ongoing system activity. As established previously, the metabolic system operates through uninterrupted redistribution, with no discrete states or fixed points. This continuous flow ensures that system state is always changing, as each adjustment modifies the configuration of substrates, signals, and constraints. The absence of static states means that context is constantly evolving, shaping how inputs are processed.

The process linking flow and context involves the continuous interaction between redistribution and state formation. As substrates are redistributed, signaling conditions adjust, and constraints interact, the system's configuration shifts incrementally. These shifts define the context in which subsequent inputs are processed, creating a feedback loop where flow influences state and state influences flow. This relationship ensures that context is always dynamic, reflecting the ongoing activity of the system.

The system implication of integrating flow and context is that there is no fixed reference point for interpretation. Each moment represents a unique configuration, shaped by prior activity and current conditions. Understanding metabolic behavior therefore requires recognizing that context is continuously changing, and that responses must be interpreted within this evolving framework.

Integration with prior mechanisms demonstrates how context governs the expression of all system behaviors. Switching efficiency varies depending on the system's configuration, influencing how smoothly transitions occur. Transition delay reflects timing misalignment that is dependent on state, with delays becoming more pronounced under certain conditions. Compensation mechanisms emerge in response to specific configurations, stabilizing the system when alignment is disrupted. Stress modifies context by altering signaling and increasing load, while electrolyte balance affects the integrity of signal transmission. Aging shapes baseline context by reducing responsiveness and increasing constraint.

The process of integrating these mechanisms involves recognizing that each operates within the context defined by system state. None of these mechanisms function independently; their expression depends on the configuration of substrates, signals, and constraints at a given moment. The outcome of any process is therefore conditional, reflecting the interaction between mechanism and context.

The system implication of this integration is that context determines how all mechanisms are expressed. Without context, the behavior of the system cannot be accurately interpreted, as the same mechanism may produce different outcomes under different conditions. This reinforces the central principle that metabolic responses are conditional, not absolute, and that meaningful interpretation requires understanding the state in which they occur.

The metabolic system therefore operates as a context-dependent process, where inputs interact with a continuously evolving state to produce outcomes. There is no meaningful interpretation of behavior without accounting for this context, as all responses reflect the integration of input and state. By recognizing context as a governing layer, the system can be understood as a dynamic and conditional process, where variability is expected and interpretation depends on the configuration in which events occur.

Flexibility as an Outcome Mechanism

Flexibility within the metabolic system is not a discrete function that can be isolated or observed independently of other processes. It emerges from the interaction of multiple mechanisms that coordinate energy redistribution across time. These mechanisms include substrate availability, signaling dynamics, transition timing, and the influence of constraints, all of which operate simultaneously. Flexibility is therefore not generated by any single pathway but arises from the alignment of these processes as they interact within the system. When coordination is maintained, flexibility appears as a property of the system's behavior rather than as a distinct action.

The process of emergence reflects how individual components contribute to a unified outcome without directly producing it. Substrate pathways adjust their contributions, signaling networks coordinate activation and suppression, and transitions occur with varying degrees of efficiency. None of these elements independently create flexibility, but their combined interaction produces a pattern of behavior that is recognized as flexible. This pattern reflects the system's capacity to redistribute energy smoothly and continuously, maintaining alignment between supply and demand across changing conditions.

The system implication of defining flexibility as an emergent property is that it cannot be understood or influenced through isolated mechanisms. Attempts to attribute flexibility to a single factor overlook the interdependence of the processes that generate it. Flexibility exists only as a reflection of coordinated system behavior, reinforcing that it is inseparable from the conditions that produce it.

Flexibility is not a direct target of the system, nor is it governed by a specific control pathway. The system does not operate with the objective of producing flexibility, and there is no mechanism that can be engaged independently to generate it. Instead, flexibility appears when the underlying processes that govern energy distribution operate in alignment. This absence of a direct control pathway distinguishes flexibility from mechanisms such as signaling or substrate mobilization, which can be described in terms of specific processes.

The process by which flexibility emerges without being targeted involves the absence of a singular point of control. Signals regulate substrate access, transitions adjust distribution, and constraints modify coordination, but none of these processes act with the explicit purpose of producing flexibility. The system responds to conditions, and flexibility arises when those responses are well-coordinated. This distinguishes flexibility from outcomes that can be directly influenced through a defined mechanism, emphasizing its dependence on overall system function.

The system implication of removing target-based framing is that flexibility cannot be approached as an objective to be achieved through direct manipulation. It is not produced by a specific action or pathway but appears when the system's processes operate cohesively. This reinforces the concept that flexibility reflects the quality of system coordination rather than the effect of any single variable.

The relationship between flexibility and stability highlights the dependence of flexible behavior on coordinated system function. Stability, defined as the continuous alignment between energy supply and demand, provides the conditions under which transitions can occur smoothly. When stability is maintained, transitions between substrates are coordinated, minimizing disruptions in energy flow. This coordination supports the expression of flexibility, as the system can adjust contributions without introducing variability.

The process linking stability to flexibility involves the synchronization of signaling, substrate availability, and transition timing. Stable systems maintain consistent communication between pathways, allowing adjustments to occur without delay or misalignment. This enables the system to redistribute energy efficiently, maintaining continuity across changing conditions. When stability is disrupted, this coordination is reduced, leading to less effective transitions and a diminished expression of flexibility.

The system implication of this relationship is that flexibility depends on the presence of stable alignment across processes. Instability introduces variability and disrupts coordination, reducing the system's capacity to maintain smooth redistribution. Flexibility therefore reflects the system's ability to sustain stability while adapting to change, rather than representing a separate capability.

Flexibility functions as a reflection of system condition, providing insight into how effectively the system's components are aligned. It reflects the combined state of signaling networks, substrate access pathways, transition dynamics, and constraint layers. These factors determine how smoothly energy is redistributed and how consistently the system maintains alignment with demand. Flexibility does not influence these components directly but represents the outcome of their interaction.

The process by which flexibility reflects system condition involves the integration of multiple variables. Signaling determines how pathways are activated, substrate access defines what resources are available, and transition quality governs how effectively redistribution occurs. Constraints such as stress, signal integrity, and aging modify these processes, influencing how they interact. The resulting behavior of the system, observed as flexibility, reflects the combined effect of these factors.

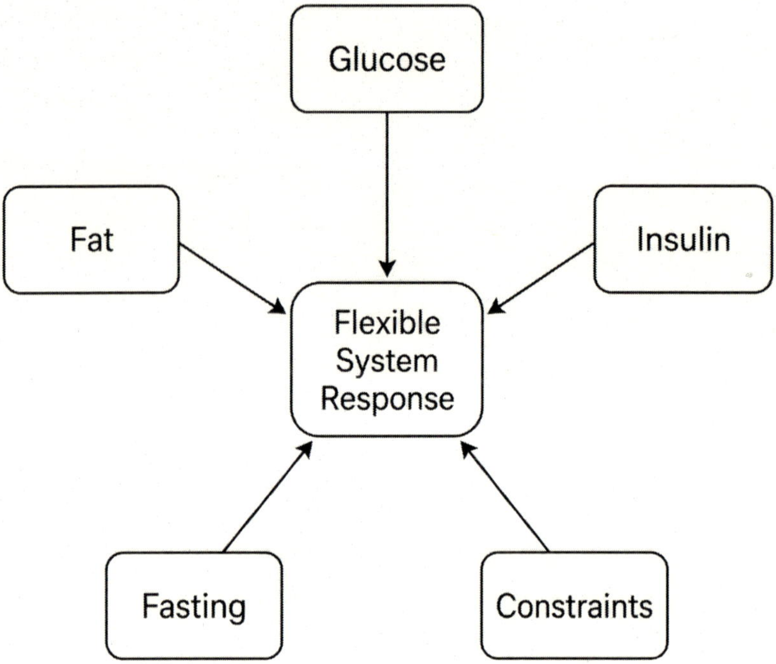

[Figure 18 — Integrated System Model]

The system implication of defining flexibility as a reflection is that it serves as an indicator of underlying system behavior rather than a driver of that behavior. Observing flexibility provides information about how well the system is functioning, but it does not explain the mechanisms that produce it. Understanding flexibility therefore requires examining the processes that contribute to it, rather than treating it as an independent variable.

The interaction of mechanisms within the system illustrates how flexibility emerges from integrated performance. Switching efficiency determines the smoothness of transitions, influencing how continuously energy is redistributed. Transition delay introduces misalignment in timing, creating interruptions in flow that affect coordination. Compensation mechanisms act to maintain continuity when alignment is disrupted, while fuel priority determines which substrates dominate under given conditions. Insulin regulates access and timing, shaping how substrates are utilized.

Stress introduces additional load, altering signaling and increasing the cost of coordination. Electrolytes influence the integrity of signal transmission, affecting how effectively pathways communicate. Aging modifies responsiveness and timing, slowing transitions and increasing the accumulation of constraints. Each of these mechanisms operates simultaneously, contributing to the system's overall behavior. Flexibility reflects the combined performance of these elements, not the action of any one component.

The system implication of multi-mechanism interaction is that flexibility cannot be attributed to individual factors. It arises from the integration of processes that influence one another, creating a network of interactions that shape system behavior. The presence or absence of flexibility reflects how well this network operates as a cohesive unit.

Constraint-limited expression explains why flexibility varies across conditions without being entirely absent. Constraints such as stress, signal degradation, and aging do not remove the system's ability to redistribute energy but modify how effectively this redistribution occurs. These constraints introduce delays, reduce coordination precision, and increase variability, limiting the expression of flexibility. The system continues to function, but its ability to maintain smooth transitions is reduced.

The process by which constraints limit flexibility involves their influence on the mechanisms that generate coordinated behavior. Stress increases signaling conflict and transition cost, while electrolyte imbalance disrupts communication between pathways. Aging slows responsiveness and extends transition duration. These factors interact to reduce the efficiency of energy redistribution, affecting the continuity of flow. Flexibility is therefore constrained rather than eliminated, reflecting the system's adjusted capacity.

The system implication of constraint-limited expression is that flexibility should be understood as a variable property that changes with system conditions. It is not present or absent in a binary sense but exists along a spectrum defined by the degree of coordination achieved. This reinforces the concept that flexibility reflects system condition rather than representing a fixed capability.

Variability in flexibility expression reflects the influence of context on system behavior. As established previously, the system operates within a continuously changing state, shaped by prior conditions, current inputs, and interacting constraints. This dynamic context influences how the mechanisms that generate flexibility are expressed, producing variation in system behavior across time. Flexibility therefore changes with context, reflecting the system's current configuration.

The process underlying variability involves the interaction between system state and the mechanisms that govern energy redistribution. Changes in signaling, substrate availability, or constraint levels alter how transitions occur, influencing the continuity of flow. These changes produce different patterns of coordination, which are observed as variations in flexibility. The system's behavior is therefore conditional, adapting to the context in which it operates.

The system implication of variability is that flexibility cannot be treated as a fixed property. It reflects the current state of the system and changes as that state evolves. Understanding flexibility requires recognizing its dependence on context, reinforcing that it is an expression of system condition rather than a stable characteristic.

Misinterpretations of flexibility often arise from attempts to associate it with specific behaviors or metrics. Observing increased use of fat as a substrate, for example, does not define flexibility, as substrate use reflects current conditions rather than overall system coordination. Similarly, conditions involving input absence do not inherently indicate flexibility, as they represent specific configurations of the system rather than its capacity for coordinated redistribution. Focusing on isolated measures reduces flexibility to a single dimension, ignoring the complexity of the processes that produce it.

The process leading to misinterpretation involves isolating one aspect of system behavior and attributing it to flexibility. This approach overlooks the role of interaction between mechanisms, treating outcomes as direct indicators rather than as context-dependent expressions. Without considering the broader system, these interpretations fail to capture the conditions that influence how flexibility is expressed. The result is an incomplete understanding of system behavior.

The system implication of removing misinterpretations is that flexibility must be evaluated as a composite outcome rather than as a single metric. No individual pathway, condition, or measure can fully represent the system's capacity for coordinated energy redistribution. Flexibility reflects the integration of multiple processes, reinforcing the need for a system-level perspective.

Integration with context dependency clarifies how flexibility is influenced by system state. As established, the same input can produce different outcomes depending on the configuration of the system. Flexibility expression follows the same principle, varying with context as the underlying mechanisms interact differently under different conditions. The system may display greater or lesser flexibility depending on how well its components are aligned within a given state.

The process linking flexibility and context involves the interaction between system condition and the mechanisms that produce coordinated behavior. Changes in state alter signaling, substrate distribution, and constraint levels, influencing how transitions occur. These changes affect the continuity of energy flow, which is observed as variation in flexibility. The system's capacity for coordinated redistribution is therefore expressed differently depending on context.

The system implication of integrating flexibility with context is that flexibility cannot be interpreted independently of system state. It reflects how the system functions under specific conditions, reinforcing that it is conditional rather than absolute. Understanding flexibility requires examining the context in which it is expressed, rather than treating it as a standalone property.

The system-level definition of flexibility emerges from integrating these principles into a unified framework. Flexibility can be defined as the system's ability to maintain coordinated energy redistribution across varying conditions. This definition emphasizes continuity, coordination, and adaptability, without reducing flexibility to specific substrates or behaviors. It reflects the system's capacity to align supply with demand while adjusting to changes in input, signaling, and constraints.

The process underlying this definition involves the interaction of all mechanisms that contribute to system function. Substrate pathways provide resources, signaling coordinates their use, transitions adjust distribution, and constraints modify how these processes interact. Flexibility reflects how effectively these elements operate together to maintain alignment across time. It is not produced by any one mechanism but emerges from their integration.

The system implication of this definition is that flexibility represents the quality of system coordination rather than a discrete function. It is expressed when the system operates in a state where its components are aligned, allowing energy to be redistributed smoothly and continuously. This reinforces the central principle that flexibility is not something the system does, but something it expresses when its processes are functioning in coordination.

Energy distribution within the system does not resolve into a final state. It remains in continuous adjustment, shaped by the interaction of availability, signaling, timing, and constraint across time. Each moment reflects a specific configuration of these factors, and each adjustment carries that configuration forward into the next. The system does not arrive at a fixed condition. It sustains alignment through ongoing coordination.

No single variable defines this behavior. Substrates, signals, transitions, and constraints do not operate independently, and outcomes do not arise from isolated causes. What is observed at any point is the result of multiple processes interacting within a given context, producing patterns that reflect the state of the system rather than the influence of any one component.

Flexibility, within this structure, is not something the system produces directly. It is the expression of coordinated interaction across these layers, appearing when alignment is maintained and diminishing when constraints limit that coordination. It reflects how the system is operating, not what it is attempting to achieve.

Understanding the system in these terms removes the need to interpret individual events as independent or definitive. Each observation exists within a continuous process, shaped by prior conditions and ongoing interactions. The system is not defined by isolated outcomes, but by the structure through which all outcomes are generated and integrated across time.

About the Author

Nathan Reed writes about metabolic stability in systems exposed to load, variability, and time.

His work examines how biological capacity is shaped by energy availability, recovery architecture, sleep amplitude, muscle mass, environmental demand and workload. Rather than treating nutrition, fasting, sleep, and training as isolated tactics, he approaches them as interacting regulatory systems governed by margin, buffering, oscillatory coherence, and constraint dominance.

The Stability framework explores how physiological compression accumulates gradually and how proportional calibration preserves long-horizon resilience across decades. The objective is not peak optimization, but preservation of functional continuity under load.

Metabolic Flexibility is part of a broader metabolic stability ecosystem developed under Perennial Publishing, each volume addressing a distinct vector of biological durability.

The work is designed for readers who prefer structural clarity over motivational rhetoric and long-horizon coherence over short-term intensity.

The Metabolic Stability Series

Metabolic Stability: *A Systems Guide to Blood Sugar, Fasting, and Long-Term Metabolic Health*

(Cornerstone Volume)

Fasting Fundamentals: *A Systems Guide to Metabolic Flexibility, Fat Loss, and Long-Term Health*

(Foundational Volume)

Intermittent Fasting: *Metabolic Timing, Body Composition, and Sustainable Health*

Prolonged Fasting: *A Systems Guide to Duration, Recovery, and Metabolic Limits*

Electrolytes: *A Systems Guide to Hydration, Electrolyte Balance, and Physiological Stability*

Insulin Stability: *Blood Sugar, Insulin Resistance, and Metabolic Health*

Glucose Stability: *How Blood Sugar Fluctuations Affect Energy, Insulin, and Metabolic Health*

Metabolic Flexibility: ***How the Body Switches Between Fat and Glucose for Energy and Metabolic Health***

Future Titles Include:

Energy Stability

Adaptation and Drift

The Vitality Series:

Sleep and Recovery

Strength and Aging

Hormones & Sexual Health

Part of a Broader Stability Framework

The Metabolic Stability Series is part of a larger stability ecosystem published by Perennial Publishing.

Related domains include:

Money Stability — structural durability in financial systems

Career Stability — positioning, load tolerance, and transition resilience

Mental Stability — cognitive steadiness under pressure and uncertainty

Emotional Stability — regulatory steadiness in environments that do not slow down

Foundations — low-fragility life architecture

Vitality — energy, strength, and biological function across time

Each domain approaches stability as a structural problem: capacity versus load, buffering versus shock, governance versus drift. Together, they form a unified framework for long-horizon durability across the major systems that shape human trajectory.

About Perennial Publishing

Perennial Publishing produces practical systems guides for building stability in an unstable world.

Our books explore the foundations of long-term resilience across health, finance, career, and everyday decision-making. Each title focuses on clear frameworks, durable principles, and practical strategies that help readers build lasting stability rather than short-term fixes.

The Perennial catalog includes series on metabolic health, financial stability, career systems, and personal consistency. While each book stands on its own, they share a common goal: helping individuals create durable systems that support a stable and sustainable life.

Made in United States
North Haven, CT
04 November 2026

21768649R00090